R
152
m42

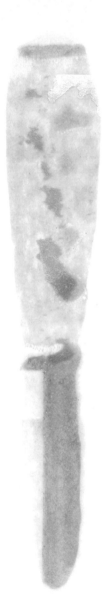

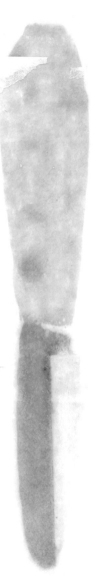

⁷8

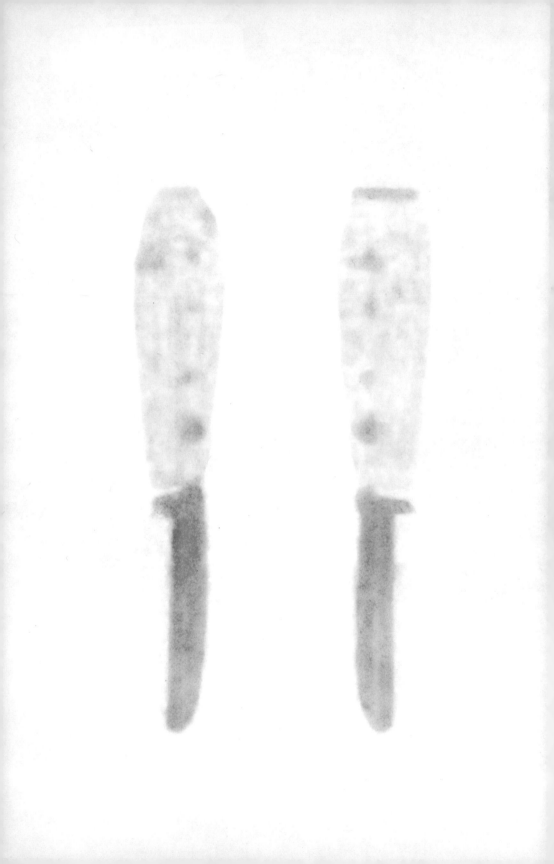

Medicine
Without
Doctors

MEDICINE WITHOUT DOCTORS

Home Health Care in American History

EDITED BY

Guenter B. Risse

Ronald L. Numbers

AND

Judith Walzer Leavitt

Science History Publications/USA

New York   1977

A Symposium organized by
the Department of the History of Medicine
University of Wisconsin, Madison

Science History Publications/USA
a division of
Neale Watson Academic Publications, Inc.
156 Fifth Avenue
New York, New York 10010

Designed and manufactured in the U.S.A.

Library of Congress Cataloging in Publication Data

Main entry under title:

Medicine without doctors.

    Includes bibliographies.
    1. Folk medicine—United States—History—
Addresses, essays, lectures. 2. Self medication—
United States—History—Addresses, essays, lectures.
I. Risse, Guenter B. II. Numbers, Ronald L.
III. Leavitt, Judith. [DNLM: 1. History of
Medicine, Modern—United States—Congresses.
2. Self medication—History—Congresses. WZ70 AA1
M4 1975]
R152.M42   615′.87882′0973   76-44943
ISBN O-88202-165-6

Contents

Illustrations

Acknowledgments

The editors would like to express their appreciation to the University of Wisconsin Medical School for its sustained financial support of the annual symposium on the history of medicine. Special thanks go to the staff of the Department of the History of Medicine, Janet Schulze Numbers, Kathryn Shain, Susan Duke, and Lawrence D. Lynch for their help in preparing the manuscripts. We are also grateful to the institutions that furnished us with illustrations, including the Library of Congress, the State Historical Society of Wisconsin, the School of Pharmacy Library of the University of Wisconsin, and the newspaper *Hospital Tribune*. Most illustrations were taken from the extensive slide collection of the Department of the History of Medicine, University of Wisconsin, Madison. Rose Jacobowitz of Neale Watson Academic Publications ably provided the finishing touches to the manuscripts. Her enthusiasm made our final task considerably easier.

Madison, January 1977

Introduction

Guenter B. Risse

"Everyone is a fool or a physician after thirty."

"He who physics himself poisons a fool."

—Proverbs

The tradition of self-help in medicine has existed since time immemorial. Until healing roles were clearly defined and professionalization was on its way, much of what constituted healing was fundamentally domestic in nature. In fact, it could be argued that healing was originally a familial or communal activity before being invested in special persons and ritualized. Individual responsibility for good health as a conscious and moral ideal to be striven for characterized the Graeco-Roman world,[1] while Christianity linked the appearance of disease to sinful actions. A sizable body of popular medical writings, largely consisting of recipes for the treatment of common complaints by laypersons, is evident from the Middle Ages onward. Herbals and so-called "Books of Secrets" provided the necessary medical and pharmacological information for successful do-it-yourself healing, especially during the sixteenth and seventeenth centuries.[2]

Eighteenth century Enlightenment writers frequently used medicine as the model for their new philosophy. They viewed medicine as an activity shedding its hitherto occult characteristics in favor of rational principles.[3] Such an optimistic outlook led to widespread hope concerning the promotion of health among the upper and middle classes. The desire to popularize medicine and make it part of the general public education gave strong impetus to the emergence of domestic literature, reflected in a series of articles in the *Encyclopédie* and the publication of books by Samuel A. Tissot (1728-1797), Bernhard C. Faust (1755-1842) and William Buchan (1729-1805).[4]

Buchan's Introduction laid down the fundamental reasons for writing such a book, which to a certain extent are still valid today.

1

First, Buchan insisted that some knowledge of medicine should be part of everybody's general education. Health education was a deterrent against quackery, facilitated better nursing and child care in the home, and contributed to a cooperative relationship with physicians. Moreover, there was in Buchan's view a demand to supply medical knowledge to "well-disposed" people, since the greater portion of the population was deprived of professional care. Finally, Buchan perceived a need to clarify and simplify available medical writings, already excessively technical and unintelligible to the layperson.

The traditional importance of do-it-yourself healing—seldom reflected in medical historiography[5]—has prompted us to examine some of its issues historically. Before proceeding further, it may be appropriate to define and describe some of the activities subsumed under medical self-help. The term broadly refers to the diagnosis, care, and even prevention of disability and illness without direct professional medical assistance. Indeed, such activity takes place most often in the privacy of one's home—hence the term *home* or *domestic* medicine. These actions can involve one's own health problems, as well as those of other family members. It must be remembered that sickness promotes a certain degree of regression and passivity, thereby creating new dependences most often involving family members and close friends. Thus, it would seem that the home is the natural setting for initially dealing with the physical and psychological effects of disease.

The next logical question relates to the nature and scope of health problems usually handled by the layperson. One obvious area for domestic medicine is minor trauma. Wound cleaning and the application of bandages is very common, and almost every household is stocked with some first-aid supplies. Another common activity is the treatment of ailments considered to be too trivial to merit professional attention. Upper respiratory conditions, gastrointestinal symptoms, mild allergic manifestations, non-specific headaches, and minor skin disorders are among the most frequently self-diagnosed and self-medicated health problems.[6]

Home medicine likewise includes nutritional measures designed to cure or aid in the convalescence from specific ailments—the so-called "invalid cookery" of yesteryear.[7] These may involve the proper feeding

2

and care of infants and children, the treatment of obesity, or the prevention of disease through proper dietary measures. If one adds the use of poultices and homemade medications derived from herbs and other eatables,[8] it is not difficult to understand another frequently employed synonym for domestic healing: *kitchen medicine.*

Finally, medical self-help includes non-professional nursing and the domestic application of hygienic principles. This may involve, for example, disinfection of rooms, insect control, and air filtration.

One of the central questions in do-it-yourself medicine is motivation. Many persons have strong feelings of self-reliance and independence which are carried over into the health care arena. Many of these attitudes are, in part, culturally conditioned and, according to some observers at least, presently on the upswing. Some people declare that they would like to have more control and power over their own lives and bodies in the face of social institutions viewed as excessively powerful and threatening to the individual. Others perceive illness as an embarrassment, an unexpected and unacceptable vulnerability subject to quick suppression with improvised home remedies.

Another important reason for practicing domestic medicine is the alleged lack of access to professional medical care, because of a scarcity of qualified medical personnel or the inability to pay for such care. Such conditions prevail in outlying rural communities as well as in urban ghettos. A case in point is the do-it-yourself medical care often employed by travelers to foreign countries where local conditions and languages create barriers to competent professional care.

A further rationale for self-healing is the real or imagined possession of certain medical knowledge on the part of the ailing individual or his advisors. To be sure, some skill in self-diagnosis and self-medication is acquired through personal experience, formal education, and exposure to popular literature and mass media advertisements. This health-related information can aid in judging the triviality of symptom–clusters and their amelioration. Most home medical manuals or encyclopedias, written by professionals, are precisely aimed at providing such basic scientific knowledge in hopes that it may actually stimulate better cooperation with health professionals.

Finally, some groups of people practice medical self-help predomi-

3

nantly because they distrust professional care. Such an attitude can be based on religious motives or the low esteem in which scientific knowledge is held. The latter reason can frequently be seen in the domestic treatment of certain chronic diseases, like arthritis, for which orthodox medicine has not yet developed a satisfactory cure—or in areas, like sexual problems, where individual professional competence is seriously doubted. Conversely, numerous conditions deemed hopeless and incurable by professionals are often treated with the unorthodox products of "kitchen medicine."

In view of the strong motivations for do-it-yourself medicine, what resources are commonly available for its practice? As already mentioned, personal and familial healing experiences are often employed to establish diagnoses and institute therapeutical actions. A sizable number of people still draw on orally transmitted folk traditions associated with their ethnic background. Thus, folklore medicine often constitutes an important ingredient of home health care.[9]

Other segments of the population rely on the sale of patent medicines and foodstuffs. Newspapers and magazines, almanacs, billboards, and mass advertising provide powerful incentives for the use of these articles, often accompanied by limited information concerning the indications for their employment. Medicine shows, public lectures, and testimonials performed the same function before the advent of cheap print and radios. Another source of information is the druggist who dispenses over-the-counter items.

Finally, the do-it-yourself public has always drawn a significant amount of medical information from physicians themselves. Publications aimed at popularizing medical knowledge have existed for centuries. This literature was, and still is, based on the assumption that a sick person knowledgeable in health matters tends to be reasonably cautious and cooperative with health professionals. Therefore, most physicians writing do-it-yourself pamphlets, books, or articles in popular magazines try to convey dietary and hygienic measures, first-aid procedures, and information concerning over-the-counter drugs. These writings also include explanations of commonly used medical terminology as well as early symptoms and signs of disease.

No activity, whether carried out by laypersons or professionals, is

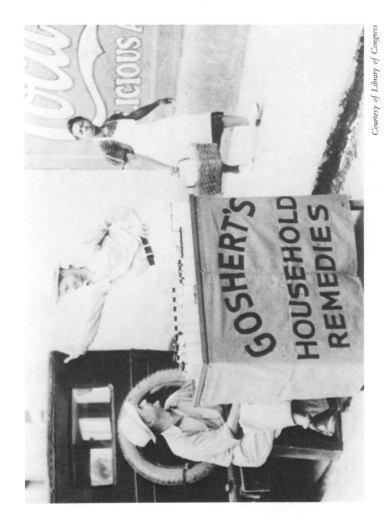

"Selling household remedies on the street, Port Gibson, Mississippi, 1940."

exempt from risks. When should self-medication be encouraged, and at what point is it desirable to seek professional attention? These are the most critical questions in the whole issue of medical self-help. The answers are frequently a function of time and judgment. In fact, the temporal duration of symptoms has been one of the most prominent factors used in deciding the above queries.

The layperson's "good" judgment is always a composite of up-to-date scientific information regarding diseases and drugs and a great deal of common sense. Nevertheless, lurking in the background are the real hazards of incorrect self-diagnosis which can delay necessary professional care. Dietary manipulations, carried out in ignorance or defiance of sound nutritional principles, can be extremely harmful. In addition, the use of home remedies by do-it-yourself healers may "mask" or suppress pathognomonic symptoms, thereby impairing the physician's subsequent ability to diagnose the illness correctly. The individual's use of unknown or untried therapeutical agents can also cause serious complications, toxicity, or possible habituation.

The papers which follow, originally delivered in April 1975 at the fourth annual symposium sponsored by the Department of the History of Medicine, University of Wisconsin, develop some of these themes. John B. Blake's survey of do-it-yourself manuals is followed by James H. Cassedy's analysis of factors that promoted American medical self-help during the first half of the nineteenth century. Ronald L. Numbers and Regina Markell Morantz discuss specific practitioners of domestic medicine: sectarians and women. James Harvey Young concludes with a description of methods employed in home medicine, especially dosing with patent medicines.

The decision to focus on the American scene—especially the last 150 years—is, of course, arbitrary. The choice was prompted primarily by the availability of sources and the existence of a nucleus of social historians of American medicine interested in the topic. Moreover, if medical self-help is an essential and possibly desirable community health resource in this country, its history should be subjected to critical examination.

Among the numerous topics remaining to be investigated are the European manuals of do-it-yourself medicine used by recently arrived immigrants. Such publications undoubtedly would illuminate some of the ethnically oriented practices which eventually succumbed to the melting process. Moreover, self-treatment among Blacks needs systematic study.

Future studies of the historical roots of medical self-help should deal in greater detail with the motivations of those laypersons who engaged in it. Class differences between patients and professional healers, therapeutic scepticism, the development of hospital medicine, and changing concepts of disease were all factors at one time or another in shaping lay attitudes toward disability and pain.

The success of the Symposium and the numerous requests received to publish the papers collectively prompt us to offer them to interested readers. We feel, however, that this book is merely a beginning toward understanding the historical role of domestic medicine. Hopefully, our efforts will spur further research in this area.

References

[1] See F. Kudlien, "The old Greek concept of 'relative' health," *J. Hist. Behavioral Sci.* 9(1973): 53-59. A view of Roman household medicine performed by the *pater familias* is contained in the writings of Pliny and Cato.

[2] J. Stannard, "Medieval herbals and their development," *Clio Medica* 9(1974): 23-33; *The Book of Secrets of Albertus Magnus*, ed. M. Best and F. Brightman (Oxford, 1973).

[3] Peter Gay, "Enlightenment: medicine and cure," in *The Enlightenment: an Interpretation* (New York: Knopf, 1969), Vol. 2, pp. 12-23.

[4] W. Coleman, "Health and hygiene in the Encyclopédie: a medical doctrine for the bourgeoisie," *J. Hist. Med.* 29(1974): 399–421; Samuel A. Tissot, *Avis au Peuple sur la Sauté* (Lausanne: Zimmerli, 1761); Bernhard C. Faust, *Gesundheits-Katechismus zum Gebrauche in den Schulen und beym hauslichen Unterrichte* (Bückeburg: Althaus, 1794); William Buchan, *Domestic Medicine* (Edinburgh: Balfour Auld and Smellie, 1769).

[5] See J.T. May, "The history of medicine and the 'crisis' in medicine," *Inquiry* 8(1971): 62-66.

[6] Mary Watkins, "Kitchen medicine," *Mother Earth News,* Des Moines, Iowa, Reprint No. 205.

[7] A small collection of recipes and old-fashioned remedies is *Grannies' Remedies,* ed. Mai Thomas (New York: Gramercy Publ. Co., 1965).

[8] Recent examples of that literature are: May Bethel, *The Healing Power of Herbs,* and Richard Lucas, *Nature's Medicines,* both published in new editions by the Wilshire Book Co. (Hollywood, California, 1974).

[9] See DeForest C. Jarvis, *Folk Medicine* (New York: Holt, 1958).

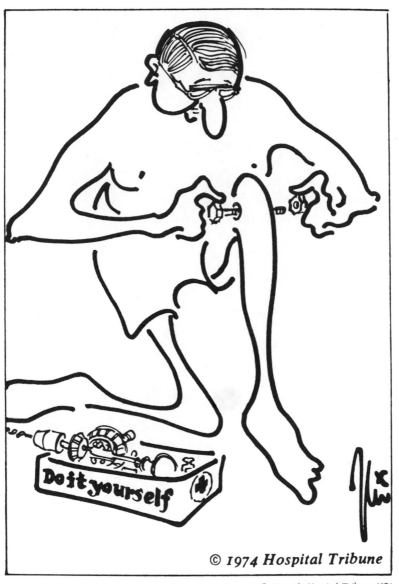

Do-it-yourself cartoon.

From Buchan to Fishbein:
The Literature of Domestic Medicine

John B. Blake

The *Modern Home Medical Adviser,* edited by Morris Fishbein, first appeared in 1935. Dr. Fishbein himself wrote on topics ranging from first aid and the family medicine chest to infectious diseases and care of the teeth. His collaborators included well-known professors from several medical schools. The book does not tell the reader how he should treat disease and injury except for emergency first aid, but informs him about disease and tells him in layman's language how physicians treat disease. It was planned, Dr. Fishbein wrote, to tell the reader "in a modern manner what every intelligent person ought to know about scientific medicine and hygiene."[1]

It has been a very successful book, reprinted often, revised, and translated; its current descendant, *The Handy Home Medical Adviser,* has sold over a million copies.[2] Books of a similar nature by equally eminent authors are widely available. Typically, the *Better Homes and Gardens Family Medical Guide* is intended, according to the introduction, to supplement the advice of one's personal physician, who alone is competent to diagnose and treat the individual. The contributors were asked to write as they would talk to their own patients if they had all the time they needed.

It is not my purpose here to examine these modern books. Suffice it to point out that they represent a flourishing form of medical literature rooted in the theme of this Symposium. By implication at least they say that self-help in medicine is best achieved by a hygienic mode of life, by some basic understanding of the human body in health and disease, and by picking a competent doctor to treat you when you are sick.

This was not always the case. In the preface to *Modern Home Medical Adviser* Dr. Fishbein described his book as "in a way a modern substitute for the old-time family medicine book that along with the Bible used to be on the table of sitting rooms in many a home in the United States." This paper will describe some of these earlier household medical books.

It is appropriate to begin with William Buchan's *Domestic Medicine.* First published in Edinburgh in 1769, it was the earliest comprehensive treatise of its kind in English. It had an immediate success, was revised and reprinted many times in America as well as Britain. A medical graduate of the University of Edinburgh, Buchan became a Fellow of the Royal College of Physicians of Edinburgh and was buried in Westminster Abbey.[3]

In the introduction to *Domestic Medicine,* Buchan argued that physicians had a duty to enlighten the public in matters relating to medicine, teaching them how to avoid disease and stay healthy through a hygienic mode of life. If people would do for themselves what they could when sick, he continued, they would rarely need to take medicines. Buchan denied any desire to teach everyone to be his own physician or to substitute his book for physicians when they could be obtained. But since half mankind could not afford doctors and it was dangerous for them to rely on quacks or charms or the rude methods of their forefathers, charitably inclined persons desirous of helping their poor neighbors should have some knowledge of proper regimen and therapeutics. They thus might also help to dispel ignorance and superstition among unlettered rustics.

Buchan devoted much attention to personal prevention of disease, including the care of children. For adults he counseled—as physicians had for centuries—a moderate, varied, and wholesome diet, temperance, fresh air, cleanliness, and exercise. He emphasized the influence of the passions on the cause and cure of diseases. He also gave some attention to diseases of occupations and social actions that would improve the public health.

In discussing diseases Buchan generally presented causes, symptoms, regimen, and medicine for each. His therapy was moderate for the time. For ague or intermittent fever, for example, despite the many "charms and whimsical remedies" that others recommended, Buchan suggested first cleansing the passages with an emetic of ipecac or a purge of Glauber's salts, jalap, or rhubarb and then concentrating on Jesuit's bark. The role of medicine was "gradually to assist nature in removing the cause of the disease." In contrast to earlier home remedy books, this represented an enlightened therapeutic outlook.[4]

Domestic Medicine:

OR, A

TREATISE

ON

THE PREVENTION AND CURE

OF

DISEASES,

BY REGIMEN AND SIMPLE MEDICINES.

WITH

An APPENDIX,

CONTAINING A DISPENSATORY FOR THE USE OF PRIVATE PRACTITIONERS.

By WILLIAM BUCHAN, M. D.

FELLOW OF THE ROYAL COLLEGE OF PHYSICIANS, EDINBURGH:

REVISED AND ADAPTED TO THE

Diseases and Climate of the United States of America,

By SAMUEL POWEL GRIFFITTS, M. D.

PROFESSOR OF MATERIA MEDICA IN THE UNIVERSITY OF PENNSYLVANIA.

PHILADELPHIA,

PRINTED BY THOMAS DOBSON,

AT THE STONE HOUSE N° 41, SOUTH SECOND-STREET.

1795.

Title page of William Buchan's *Domestic Medicine,* first American edition, 1795.

Not long after the Revolution, American physicians, no doubt impressed by their new independence with a sense of the special character of American diseases as well as other American institutions, began issuing new editions of Buchan "revised and adapted," according to the title page of one, "to the diseases and climate of the United States." The editor, Dr. Samuel P. Griffitts of the University of Pennsylvania, added a chapter on yellow fever and occasional notes on American practice. For example, Buchan had noted that in inflammation of the liver, bleeding was proper, but that all violent purgatives were to be avoided; if necessary the body might be kept gently open by a decoction of tamarinds with honey or manna. In a footnote Griffitts pointed out that the American practice, after bleeding and purging, was to give two to three grains of calomel twice a day and inunctions of mercurial ointment until the disease was subdued. The fears that some had of the "rough and inflammatory nature" of calomel, he wrote elsewhere, were "totally groundless." Considering that it was the cathartic almost universally used for children, it could hardly be thought to be too strong for adults.[5]

By 1826, Anthony Benezet, a medical graduate of the University of Pennsylvania residing in Cincinnati, had decided that a more thorough-going Americanization of Buchan was called for. In a work entitled *The Family Physician,* "calculated particularly for the inhabitants of the western country, and for those who navigate its waters," Benezet freely acknowledged his indebtedness to Buchan's "valuable treatise." He was, wrote Benezet, "a philanthropist, as well as an able Physician." However, improvements in medicine since his day, and the differences in climate between his country and America, had rendered much of his work obsolete or useless so far as it pertained to the treatment of disease. Benezet's recital of the reasons why such books were needed was also Americanized. While acknowledging that "in every important case of disease, a skilful medical man . . . ought to be employed," this was not always possible. Many American practitioners unfortunately, especially in remote places, from want of opportunity were inadequately trained, and quacks abounded. Public enlightenment in the medical art would help to solve this problem. Benezet does not suggest that inability to pay was an important consideration nor does he propose his book as a guide to the charitably inclined. Such motives evidently seemed out of place in the self-reliant American West.

Benezet's Americanization also showed in his advice to immigrants on seeking a healthy location. Especially does it appear in his therapeutics. Simple nourishment and avoidance of stimulants was fine for those in health, but when the body became disordered, he wrote, "'the work,' to borrow a phrase of Dr. Rush, 'must be taken out of nature's hands.'" In Benezet's view, "Mildness of medical treatment is real cruelty." In this respect Buchan's and most other books of domestic medicine were wrong; only lately and in the United States had physicians become convinced of the need for a "decisive, prompt, and vigorous mode of practice; the diseases of our own country," wrote Benezet, "especially require it." Thus, in treating intermittent fever, this author called first for evacuating the stomach and bowels with 8 grains of tartar emetic in a half pint of water taken 2 tablespoons at a time every 15 minutes; followed "as soon as the patient appears able to bear it" by a purge of 15 grains of calomel plus 25 grains of Epsom salts. These might be taken, he assured, "with perfect safety." Later, tonics were proper: Peruvian bark was a powerful one and useful, though its specific virtues were doubtful; some might wish to try the new drug, quinine. Benezet was rather partial to an infusion of quassia wood in wine with Fowler's solution of arsenic added. In serious cases of the more severe bilious fever, Benezet had administered 100 grains of calomel combined with 8 grains of opium in pills of 4 grains each over a period of 16 hours.[6]

Benezet's work is in many ways typical of those written by regular physicians in the early decades of the nineteenth century. Characteristically they claimed to be intended for persons who could not obtain the services of a physician because they were isolated in the country or on a ship at sea, or for planters to treat their slaves. Emphasis was placed on the value of the books in teaching the public how to avoid quacks and empirics whose pretensions were fostered by public ignorance, with the hope that this would also increase their appreciation for a true physician and his treatments. Thus Thomas Ewell, also a medical graduate of Pennsylvania, in his *American Family Physician,* published in Georgetown, D.C., in 1824, expressed the view that it was much better for physicians to practice in families that knew something about medicine. They would be more likely to call the physician promptly when sick and to follow his directions.[7] Similarly, Thomas W. Ruble, M.D., in *The American Medical Guide for the Use of Families,* published in Richmond, Kentucky, in 1810, explained that his greatest difficulty came from his patients' ignorance and superstition. But after explaining and justifying his prescriptions, he generally was able to reconcile the family "to the use of some of the most powerful drugs of the shops, at the very name of which they would at first shuder [sic]," so that "many families now deal out opium, mercury, tartar, &c. with a liberal hand, that once would have turned pale at the very name." For Ruble, calomel was "a gentle purgative" excellent for worms in children and tartar emetic a "sovereign febrifuge."[8] Such heroic practice is also characteristic of these books, well into the 1850s.

Already, however, other physician-authors of domestic medical books had begun to pay more than lip service to the view that people should call in the doctor for serious problems rather than treating themselves. Thomas Cooper's *Treatise of Domestic Medicine,* published in Reading, Pennsylvania, in 1824, consisted chiefly of a variety of injuries, diseases, and symptoms arranged alphabetically, with directions. But frequently the only direction is "Apply to a physician," or "Send for a surgeon." Dr. Cooper advised families living in the country to keep on hand castor oil, Epsom salts, calomel, jalap, tartar emetic, ipecac, and a number of other drugs, but no lancet, opium, or laudanum, "for they are too dangerous to be trusted to unskilful persons." Cooper's work is also notable for some decidedly unusual comments on the subject of alcoholic beverages:

> I have travelled the circuit for five and twenty years, as lawyer and judge, and have had occasion and temptation, to drink all sorts of wine, and all qualities, moderately and sometimes immoderately; and therefore consider myself qualified to speak of it. . . . The pleasantest wines are in this order,—Burgundy of Romanne-Conty, Claret of La Fitte, Chateau-Margaut, or medoc generally: but no claret, is drinkable for pleasure or health, except the first quality.[9]

Dr. William Matthews's *Treatise on Domestic Medicine,* printed in Indianapolis in 1848, moved still further away from the heroic self-reliance of most of his predecessors. Perhaps influenced by the growing health reform movement, he devoted nearly a quarter of his small book to the anatomy and physiology of the normal human body and to hygiene. More important he introduced a new therapeutic attitude. "Now, it is the tendency of many diseases to cure themselves," he wrote, "or rather to be cured by the unaided efforts of the constitution." The medical man must be able to recognize these cases, gently assist nature when necessary, and refrain from officious interference. Specifically, he acknowledged that although an emetic of ipecac and a purge of castor oil might be useful in intermittent fever, the important thing was large doses of quinine during the intermission. In bilious remittent fever, where his predecessors had urged massive doses of calomel, Matthews stated that purges and emetics were often improper; his advice was to call a physician. "The public are too fond of taking medicine," he wrote, "and are apt to attribute too much to its curative influence. Medicine, like every thing else, is good in its place, but it is not always, and under all circumstances, good to make Apothecaries' Shops of people's stomachs!" Most unusual, perhaps, was Matthews's acknowledgment that consumption, once "firmly fixed upon the lungs," was incurable, and that the physician's task was to smooth the path to the grave.[10]

Competing with the books that have been described, from the time of Buchan's or earlier, were others quite different in character. Instead of suggesting that they be used only in the absence of a physician, many books of domestic medicine consciously attacked the regular profession and argued in effect that every man should be his own physician. One of the most influential and long-lived was the Methodist John Wesley's *Primitive Physick*. First published in London in 1747, it was reprinted in Philadelphia in 1764 and continued popular in America until well into the nineteenth century. Originally, according to Wesley, cures were empirical discoveries passed down from father to son, suited to the climate and available natural products of a particular region. But then men began to inquire into the causes of things. Discarding "experiment" and simple medicines, they began to prescribe according to theory, and physic became an abstruse science out of the reach of ordinary men. When physicians found that this raised their status and enhanced their profits, they designedly increased the number of exotic drugs and the mystery surrounding medicine, while branding as empirics those who knew only how to restore the sick to health. His book, Wesley wrote, would return medicine to its primitive simplicity, when there was no need for anatomy or natural philosophy, but only the knowledge that "Such a Medicine removes such a Pain." Thus one could have a physician always in the home to prescribe without fee, and multitudes could be saved from pining away in sickness and pain through the ignorance or knavery of physicians. The book would provide only cheap and safe medicines easily procured and easily applied by plain, unlettered men: but no antimony, opium, bark, steel, or mercury (although there are in fact a few recipes using some of these drugs). Generally Wesley followed the old cookbook pattern of naming a disease, symptom, or injury and following it with several prescriptions, mostly herbal simples. Occasionally a line or two is added to describe the disease.[11]

Like Wesley in his contempt for the regular medical profession was the well-known native American original, Samuel Thomson. Thomson created and then patented a new "system" of medicine, which all might use who purchased the rights. Thomsonians were among the most effective and successful opponents of licensing laws for physicians, attacking them for their anti-democratic monopolistic privileges. As the movement gained ground, Thomson lost control and the trappings of a profession—special schools, societies, conventions, and so on—took over.[12] But other writers carried forward the notion that medicine was basically a simple business that everyone should be able to handle for himself. Thus, Samuel North in his *Family Physician and Guide to Health,* published in Waterloo, New York, in 1830, sounding not unlike Wesley, complained that medical writers "from a plentiful use of technical terms and scraps of obsolete latin . . . have not only made their works unintelligible to general readers, but impressed the minds of the multitude with a proper respect for the unfathomable arcana of medicine. . . ." His purpose was to enable "men of common capacities" to administer "simple, easy, and cheap" remedies. Like Wesley also, North offered many different suggested treatments for various disorders. His sources were eclectic, ranging from Tissot to Thomson and the Indians.[13]

North's fellow New Yorker, Dr. Daniel H. Whitney, author of

The Family Physician, and Guide to Health, thought people should no more need send to a physician to know what medicine to take than to a butcher to know what meat to eat.

> I have always been surprised to see people look with so much confidence to the physician, in cases of imminent danger, and place so much stress upon the necessity of his presence, when all that he was doing or could do, was to give an emetic perhaps, or a dose of calomel. . . . the practice of medicine is not of half the consequence that it is generally imagined to be.[14]

Among the plethora of nineteenth century domestic medical works, one of the most popular was J.C. Gunn's *Domestic Medicine, or Poor Man's Friend.* First published in Knoxville in 1830, it reached the so-called 100th edition (now titled *Gunn's New Family Physician; or Home Book of Health*) in 1870, and was still going strong. Combining nationalism, anti-intellectualism, and piety, Gunn made note in early editions that professional pride and cupidity had delighted in concealing the art of healing. But God in his mercy had "stored our mountains, fields and meadows, with simples for healing our diseases," making foreign drugs, often adulterated or expensive, unnecessary. The learned, Gunn complained, used words "to conceal the naked poverty and bareness of the sciences. . . . if the great mass of the people knew how much pains were taken by scientific men, to throw dust in their eyes by the use of ridiculous and high-sounding terms . . . mankind would soon be undeceived, as to the little difference that really exists between themselves and the *very learned* portion of the community." Hypocrisy in religion, pettifogging in law, and quackery in medicine were being dispersed by the progress of knowledge; people were learning that once the fancy language was eliminated, the sciences became common sense, easily understood by all.

It was Gunn's purpose, of course, to reduce the practice of medicine to common sense. For all his talk of the products of American forests and fields, Gunn's actual practice was often not far different from that of the regulars. Bilious fever, he wrote, though a "formidable and dangerous disease, may in most instances be easily subdued, if you will divest yourself of irresolution and timidity in the commencement of the attack." He recommended tartar emetic to cleanse the stomach,

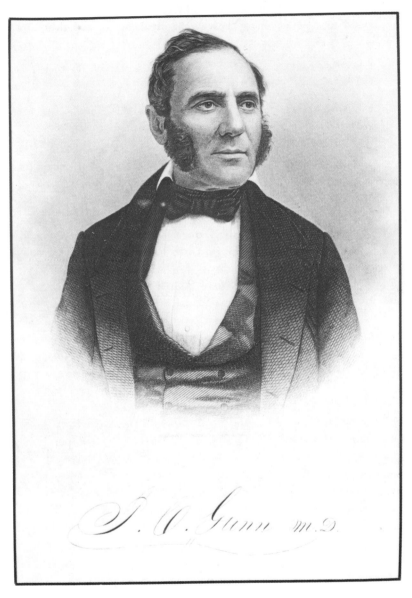

Portrait of John Gunn,
frontispiece of *Gunn's New Domestic Physician*, 1862.

GUNN'S

NEW DOMESTIC PHYSICIAN:

OR

HOME BOOK OF HEALTH,

A COMPLETE GUIDE FOR FAMILIES,

POINTING OUT IN FAMILIAR AND PLAIN TERMS THE CAUSES, SYMPTOMS, TREATMENT
AND CURE OF THE DISEASES INCIDENT TO

MEN, WOMEN AND CHILDREN,

WITH DIRECTIONS FOR USING

MEDICINAL PLANTS

AND THE SIMPLEST AND BEST

NEW REMEDIES,

AND GIVING ALSO

MANY VALUABLE RULES FOR AVOIDING DISEASE AND PROLONGING LIFE.

BY JOHN C. GUNN, M.D.,

AUTHOR OF "GUNN'S DOMESTIC MEDICINE."

WITH AN APPENDIX ON

ANATOMY, PHYSIOLOGY, Etc., Etc.

CINCINNATI:
MOORE, WILSTACH, KEYS & CO.,

No. 25 WEST FOURTH STREET.

SAN FRANCISCO: NIMAN & BOALS.

GENERAL AGENTS FOR CALIFORNIA AND OREGON.

1862.

SOLD TO SUBSCRIBERS ONLY.

Title page of John Gunn's *New Domestic Physician,*
1862.

bleeding freely, and 20 grains each of calomel and jalap—repeated, if necessary, by another dose of 30 grains. It was the administration of small, 8 to 10 grain doses, in Gunn's opinion, that had brought disgrace to the use of calomel in recent years. Gunn's attitude toward surgery was equally heroic: any man with firmness and common dexterity, he wrote, could amputate a limb. His contemporary A.G. Goodlett made it seem even simpler: in his *Family Physician* of 1838 he promised to explain amputation so that "any man, unless he is an idiot or an absolute fool, can perform this operation."[15]

Writers like Gunn and Goodlett attacked the alleged mumbo-jumbo of doctors and professed to make medicine plain and easy for all, but their therapeutics were more or less standard. Still other types of domestic medicine books did not so much attack the learned physician as ignore him. Most of these consist largely of collections of recipes, often intermingling those for the cure of various diseases with various household receipts and farriery. Eighteenth century cookbooks often included material of this type,[16] and Wesley's *Primitive Physick* was largely a collection of recipes, though his conscious attack on doctors puts the work in a separate category. Rather more old-fashioned than Wesley in spirit, though much later, was *The Treasure of Health* published by Lewis Merlin in 1819. It purported to be "a wonderful collection of the most valuable secrets in medicine, for the cure of all diseases, wounds, and other accidents to which the human body is subject." It was a typical book of secrets, such as were common 200 years before, containing never-failing recipes for treating (incurable) diseases, at least one of which was credited to Queen Elizabeth of England.[17]

In republican America more plebeian literature soon took over. The tendency is readily seen in an edition of Buchan's *Domestic Medicine* published in New Haven in 1816. Retitled *Every Man His Own Doctor,* it omits most of Buchan's prefatory material explaining the rationale of the book and adds a treatise on farriery and a "Universal Receipt Book." The first four receipts are a cure for jaundice, the German method of clarifying and preserving butter, lozenges for heartburn, and a catsup that would keep for 20 years.[18]

A few years later, Josiah Richardson compiled *The New England Farrier, and Family Physician* (Exeter, 1828), including a wide variety of household, medical, and what Richardson called "brutal" receipts. One of the last, "for a creature choaked," starts out, "Take one cartridge of gun powder . . ." Emptied down the poor brute's throat, "it will effect an immediate cure." The medical receipts were equally crude. Thus:

> *To cure the asthma.* Take the bag that holds the musk of a skunk, and hang it up in the room where the person lives—rub it about the mouth and nose, smelling of it often—if very bad, take two or three drops of the musk, or more, as you need. This has given great relief, so that the speechless have been relieved, and have got well.

For fever and ague, Richardson recommended a decoction of horsemint, mullein root, stinkweed root, and red pepper pods. A collection of receipts attributed to "a learned, pious & skilful English physician" which Richardson included turns out to be largely—of all things— a reprint of Wesley's *Primitive Physick.*[19] Similar collections of health and household recipes continued popular for years to come, not only in books but also in almanacs, newspapers, and similar forms of popular literature.

Even without counting advertising publications, it is evident that family medical books were very popular. The ones cited in this paper represent only a small portion of the total production, and many went through repeated "editions" or reprintings. Obviously they were perceived to meet a need. During much of the nineteenth century it was difficult for many rural families to get a doctor. They lived, often, in isolation, roads were poor, travel slow, sickness prevalent, emergencies many. Doctors could be expensive, too, for a farming family with a very small cash income.

Many of the books also appealed to current American prejudices in other ways. The earlier ones especially played on nationalism by emphasizing that they were written for American climate and diseases. Later, in an era of Know-Nothingism, there were those that touted native products, usually herbal, as an alternative to expensive and probably adulterated foreign imports. The idea that God would provide in America the necessary means to cure diseases found in America, an argument once used to promote the sale of guaiac for the treatment of syphilis, added piety to nationalism. Religion was also brought in by those authors who attributed disease among mankind to Adam's first sin, and by others when discussing the passions.

Many authors, by attacking the regular medical profession or declaring special training unnecessary, catered to the anti-monopoly, sometimes anti-intellectual, common-man democracy of the Jacksonian era, and the low opinion of physicians held by much of the public. Hence we also find that special virtues were often attributed to Indian medicine, particularly by those who were anti-calomel. Considering the training of some who held the M.D. degree, it was perhaps not too farfetched to argue that anyone could do as well by perusing a book or two, and the increase in common schooling during the nineteenth century enlarged the percentage of those able to read and therefore the market for books. Finally it must be remembered that guides for self-treatment were neither new in the nineteenth century nor specifically American. Popular medicine is ancient history.

The trend away from home treatments in books by members of the regular medical profession, seen in a few works before the Civil War, was carried further by George M. Beard, an author best known for his works on neurasthenia, in *Our Home Physician,* published in New York in 1869. Besides the other usual objectives—preventing disease by teaching a healthy way of life and providing instructions for emergency first aid or for persons beyond the reach of a doctor—Beard emphasized the value of knowledge for its own sake. His aim, he wrote, was to say "just what the family physician would tell his patients if he had the time and strength to give instruction in science to the families under his charge." He strongly favored efforts to popularize scientific and medical knowledge, partly on grounds that it would enable members of the public to perform their civic duties more intelligently, arguing that the habit of looking at things from a scientific point of view was necessary if the country was to solve its many social and political problems. The widespread scientific ignorance prevailing in the United States was deplorable: legislatures, judges, clergy, and other leaders were called upon to decide matters relating to science that they knew nothing about. Beard attacked not only quacks and charlatans, but food faddists like Sylvester Graham and William A. Alcott for their erroneous and unscientific views, though Beard himself suffered from a number of nationalistic as well as dietary prejudices. "Potato diet, when exclusive," he wrote, "makes potato brains. Witness the Irish peasantry."[20]

In 1880 *Wood's Household Practice of Medicine, Hygiene and Surgery,* edited by Frederick A. Castle, similarly emphasized the desirability of general public knowledge of health and disease as well as specific knowledge for emergencies and a limited number of minor ills. The work eliminated most of the kind of information still available in Beard's which might tempt the public to treat themselves for serious, non-emergency conditions. Like many of its successors it included contributions from a number of distinguished authors. Quite clearly more physicians were accepting the view set forth in the preface that they had a duty to enlighten the public, particularly on means to avoid disease. Comparable works appeared later with some regularity. *The Home Medical Library* published in 1907 included contributions by Thomas Darlington, Commissioner of Health for New York City, and S. Weir Mitchell. Thus Dr. Fishbein's *Modern Home Medical Adviser,* appearing in 1935, reinforced a trend already well established.

From Buchan in 1769 to Fishbein in 1935, domestic medicine books written by regular physicians had advanced from simplified textbooks of medical practice for those who could not obtain the services of a physician with, usually, some rules of hygiene, to informational or educational books about health and disease, with the do-it-yourself aspects strictly limited to hygiene and emergency first aid. In the process, they also mirrored changes in medical science and practice itself.

Some reasons for this shift may be suggested. As the population expanded and the country became more settled and farms less isolated, the need for self-treatment declined. As the nation became more urban and industrial, the remaining demand for self-treatment could be more easily filled by the ever growing patent medicine industry. During the nineteenth century, medicine had become in many ways more complex. It was easier to write for the layman when the most important diseases of general concern were to be treated by tartar emetic and calomel, with an occasional bow to Peruvian bark. As the century progressed, this therapeutics became unacceptable, and especially outside of the

South the intermittent and remittent bilious fevers no longer played so dominant a role among the diseases of rural America.

Physicians, too, were becoming better educated and less ready to suggest that there was a cure for every disease, or that every man could be his own physician. The increasing success and new discoveries of medicine toward the end of the century muted attacks on the profession. An increased demand and need for public enlightenment and education in the sciences was perceived and a number of popularizers were attempting both to foster and to meet it. If doctors did not accept a public responsibility to teach health and hygiene, others would. "Oh, hygiene," wrote one, "how many crimes have been committed in thy name!"[21] The need and responsibility for public education still exist.

References

[1] Morris Fishbein, ed., *Modern Home Medical Adviser* (New York: Doubleday, Doran, 1935), preface.

[2] Personal communication.

[3] For a recent discussion of Buchan, see C.J. Lawrence, "William Buchan: medicine laid open," *Medical History,* 19(1975):20-35. The general subject of this paper has previously been considered in L.S. King, "Do-it-yourself medicine," *Journal of the American Medical Association,* 200(1967):23-29. Several of the works are also described in M.E. Pickard and R.C. Buley, *The Midwest Pioneer: His Ills, Cures & Doctors* (Crawfordsville, Ind.: R.E. Banta, 1945), pp. 89-95.

[4] William Buchan, *Domestic Medicine; or, The Family Physician* (Philadelphia: R. Aitken, [1771]), pp. iii-vi, 1-91, 103-107.

[5] William Buchan, *Domestic Medicine; or, A Treatise on the Prevention and Cure of Diseases, by Regimen and Simple Medicines,* rev. Samuel Powel Griffitts (Philadelphia: T. Dobson, 1795), title page, pp. 223, 314-315. Another adaptation of Buchan's book, by Isaac Cathrall, published 1797, followed essentially the same line.

[6] Anthony A. Benezet, *The Family Physician; Comprising Rules for the Prevention and Cure of Diseases; Calculated Particularly for the Inhabitants of the Western Country, and for Those Who Navigate Its Waters* (Cincinnati: W.H. Woodward, 1826), pp. 3-9, 15-29, 106, 108-113.

[7] Thomas Ewell, *American Family Physician; Detailing Important Means of Preserving Health, from Infancy to Old Age* (Georgetown, D.C.: J. Thomas, 1824), pp. xi-xii.

[8] Thomas W. Ruble, *The American Medical Guide for the Use of Families* (Richmond, Ky.: E. Harris, 1810), pp. iii-iv, 24, 84.

[9] Thomas Cooper, *A Treatise of Domestic Medicine* (Reading, Pa.: G. Getz, 1824), pp. 2, 5.

[10] William Matthews, *A Treatise on Domestic Medicne* [sic] *and Kindred Subjects: Embracing Anatomical and Physiological Sketches of the Human Body* (Indianapolis: J.D. Defrees, 1848), pp. 36-37, 54-56, 59, 65-66, 86.

[11] John Wesley, *Primitive Physick: or, an Easy and Natural Method of Curing Most Diseases* 12th ed. (Philadelphia: A. Steuart, 1764), pp. iii–xviii; recipes no. 300, 328, 450, 694, 759, 760, 769. See G.S. Rousseau, "John Wesley's *Primitive Physic* (1747)," *Harvard Library Bulletin* 16(1968): 242–256.

[12] Thomson's career is described in Dr. Numbers's paper in this Symposium.

[13] Samuel North, *The Family Physician and Guide to Health, Together with Some Remarks on Surgery* (Waterloo, N.Y.: Wm. Child, 1830) pp. iii–iv and *passim.*

[14] Daniel H. Whitney, *The Family Physician, and Guide to Health* (Penn-Yan, N.Y.: H. Gilbert, 1833), pp. iii–iv.

[15] John C. Gunn, *Gunn's Domestic Medicine, or Poor Man's Friend, in the Hours of Affliction, Pain and Sickness* 4th ed. (Madisonville: Henderson & Johnston, 1834), pp. xi–xii, 97, 147–148, 564; A.G. Goodlett, *The Family Physician, or Every Man's Companion* (Nashville, Tenn.: Smith and Nesbit, 1838), p. 622.

[16] J.B. Blake, "The compleat housewife," *Bulletin of the History of Medicine* 49(1975):30–42.

[17] Lewis Merlin, *The Treasure of Health* (Philadelphia, 1819), title page, p. 222, and *passim.*

[18] William Buchan, *Every Man His Own Doctor; or, A Treatise on the Prevention and Cure of Diseases, by Regimen and Simple Medicines* (New Haven: N. Whiting, 1816), part 2, pp. 87–88.

[19] Josiah Richardson, compiler, *The New-England Farrier, and Family Physician* (Exeter: J. Richardson, 1828), pp. 45, 65–66, 70, 155–232.

[20] George M. Beard, *Our Home Physician: A New and Popular Guide to the Art of Preserving Health and Treating Disease* (New York: E.B. Treat, 1869), pp. iii–xxi, 167, 194.

[21] J.M. Tyler, "The responsibility of the physician for public education in physiology and hygiene," *Bulletin of the American Academy of Medicine* 11(1910):688–691.

Why Self-Help?
Americans Alone with their Diseases
1800–1850

James H. Cassedy

Throughout our history and down to the present, American viewpoints toward the use of physicians and disease therapies have been about as diverse as the population itself. Some Americans, of course, have habitually deferred to the professional expertise of the medical profession. Others have tended to regard themselves as being fully as competent as the physician. Most have doubtless sought out physicians for their serious illnesses. However, few can have found any need to consult a physician for their myriads of minor scratches, headaches, or insect bites. In fact, wherever people have been able to obtain their own medicines, or have read books about hygiene, or have had relatives, neighbors, or travellers to suggest remedies, they have been ready in large numbers to rely on such sources and on their own judgments rather than resort to physicians even with serious ailments.

Individuals in this country as elsewhere have resorted to medical self-care for various important but largely intangible reasons, including personal inertia or convenience, well-established family or social habits, and the influence of strongly held individual or group principles. However, there have also been powerful external factors which made self-help a necessity and which helped shape Americans' overall attitudes toward the practice. Among these have been the geographical isolation of potential medical consumers, the expense of medical care, and the inadequate supply or performance of the medical profession. This paper will focus upon some of these determinants.

It is possible to maintain, at least for argument's sake, that most people, at most stages of American history, lived close enough to a medically trained individual that they could usually obtain his services when they really needed these. Let me pursue this argument briefly. It is undeniably true that there were some physicians, together with other professional men, serving the larger centers of population from the earliest days of settlement. Over the decades, as the towns grew into cities, more and more physicians came to this country from Europe, and formal facilities to train doctors began to develop here, while at the same time there was a steady accumulation of medical institutions—quarantine stations, medical societies, hospitals, clinics, medical journals, and other appurtenances of the physician. Viewed in the aggregate, all of this readily suggests that health was being taken care of, that the medical profession was growing at about the same pace as the general population, that the ordinary man was reasonably well provided with professional medical attention.

To press the argument a little further, one can point to a long history of expedients which have been adopted in America to bring medical attention even to those living outside the centers of population. During the early periods this meant essentially the services of itinerants. In the mid-seventeenth century, we recall, Governor John Winthrop, Jr., carried medical knowledge and care out to hundreds of settlers along the coasts and rivers of Connecticut as he made the rounds of his colony. And, a hundred years later, physicians like John Mitchell made their medical circuits of the scattered plantations of tidewater Virginia. A well-known popular work has gone on to glorify this American tradition of "doctors on horseback" of the late eighteenth and early nineteenth centuries, even though four of its seven main figures were essentially urban practitioners.[1] And the twentieth century has made its own grand efforts—with its health trains, visiting nurses, emergency helicopters, and communication satellites—to bring medical care to outlying areas of the United States.

Perhaps, on the strength of the expanding numbers of physicians, medical institutions, and medical expedients, we can accept the view that most people of the past two or three hundred years have found some, more or less professional, medical care available. But this view of an indeterminate and perhaps hypothetical majority does not account for those who may not have taken advantage of such care even when it was readily available. And even more important, it leaves out an equally indeterminate, but for some periods sizable, minority of people who for some reason found themselves involuntarily alone medically when confronted with assorted serious fevers, epidemics, and accidental injuries. We are primarily interested here in the predicament of such individuals as a stimulus to home doctoring.

During the seventeenth and eighteenth centuries, whole towns and villages sometimes found themselves in this predicament, without any professional medical care available and presumably without even a clergyman who knew any medicine. Some towns attempted to alleviate the situation by petitioning or advertising for a physician to settle in their communities, and doubtless many others should have. Individuals who pushed very far out of towns that did have physicians could find an abundance of land, but in so doing they not infrequently found themselves outside the feasible orbit of the local doctors' visits. Up into our own times, the remoteness of medical facilities has remained a frequent disadvantage for rural inhabitants. And realistic writers from Edward Eggleston to Hamlin Garland and Ole Rolvaag have suggested something of the periodic medical pains and tragedies of that life. In the early 1920s, the muckraker Samuel Hopkins Adams found rural medical services actually declining rather than increasing. The old-time country doctor was vanishing, and younger physicians were increasingly being drawn into practice in urban areas. As Adams wrote: "They would rather starve in the cities, where scientific and social advantages are available, than make an assured living in the country." And this dilemma was being further accelerated and complicated, Adams saw, by the rise of medical specialization, which flourished best in the urban context.[2]

Such conditions, where trained medical care has been unavailable or inaccessible, clearly were among those which have driven the potential American medical consumer in every century to the quack, the irregular physician, the patent medicine shelf of the drugstore, to a variety of home medical expedients, or to the point of rejecting doctors and medicines. In the remainder of this paper I want to examine in somewhat greater detail how these and related factors contributed to the practice of self-medication over a more limited time span, namely the first half of the nineteenth century.

It was no secret to anyone, in mid-nineteenth century, that Americans were exceedingly eclectic in their medical habits. Members of the regular medical profession, of course, were painfully aware of the large numbers of the sick who resorted to self-medication expedients rather than seeking professional advice and treatment. While many such physicians banded together, particularly in the new American Medical Association, to try to resist some of these tendencies, others tried to gather evidence which might show the medical consequences of alternate forms of care. Samuel Cartwright claimed that the mortality in Natchez, Mississippi, during the 1830s, increased drastically with the arrival of and widespread use of steam doctors and quacks. The New Englander William A. Alcott, on the other hand, was particularly concerned with the huge extent of infant mortality caused by "maternal dosing and drugging." He had found that "the vast majority of our mothers doctor . . . their own children . . . [with] a vast amount of small elixirs, cordials, &c," and most did it with little knowledge of the effects.

In St. Louis, J.V. Prather went somewhat further into the bad consequences which he believed were caused by the medical habits of his fellow townsmen. During the 1840s he found that heavy child mortality was resulting partly from a reliance on quacks and irregular doctors, but even more from self-medication and a failure to use any kind of doctor. Over a four-month period in 1847, 469 deaths were reported of children five years old or younger. Of these, Prather found that only 133 were known to have been under the care of regular physicians. Of the rest, 100 had been treated by quacks or irregulars, 31 by unknown means, and 205 by no physician at all. Prather ventured to suggest a number of reasons for this widespread tendency not to use physicians: a preference for old wives' recipes and other home prescriptions, frequent switching of physicians, a general "love for new things or remedies," and the "fear of expense." He might also have noted some further causes that reflected on the medical profession itself: organized medicine's lack of authority throughout this period, its lack of certain knowledge about disease and therapy, the demoralizing and divisive controversialism which had long been epidemic among physicians. These conditions alone were prominent among the causes of doubt which contributed to the substantial self-medication of the nineteenth century. They should be kept in mind in connection with the problem of the supply of medical men.[3]

Although there were other sources of new doctors, the most prominent factor in physician supply during these years was the network of native medical schools. Between 1790 and 1850, of course, these schools multiplied rapidly. In fact, the increase from three schools to thirty-five, not counting the emergence of sectarian institutions, was a rough reflection of the growth in population, which rose from some 3,900,000 to about 23,200,000. There was also an apparent substantial increase in the proportion of physicians to the population—from somewhere between one in 800 and one in 1100 in 1790, to roughly one in 570 in 1850. In numbers this was a rise from somewhere between 3,500 and 4,900 in 1790, to the 40,564 physicians who were enumerated in the census of 1850.[4]

Statistically, of course, this growth suggests a very favorable state of affairs for the American medical consumer, particularly as the number of some 40,000 physicians for 1850 probably did not include most of the assorted irregular practitioners of the day. But for the regular medical profession, the enormous increase created enormous problems. In fact, as early as the late 1830s, the uncontrolled proliferation of proprietary schools was a matter of great concern. The adverse effect that this situation had on the quality of medical education was one problem. The newly controversial role of medical schools as profit-seeking institutions was another. Charles Caldwell, noting this "medical school mania" in 1834, thought that four such institutions instead of the twenty that had already appeared were quite enough at that time, and, in the long run, one school for every four or five million people instead of the current one for every seven or eight hundred thousand. During the next several decades, establishment physicians by the dozens—men like Caldwell who had financial stakes in some medical school or other—went into print to deplore the establishment of new competing schools. But others, who had no such stakes, were troubled primarily by what appeared to be an unabsorbable surplus of physicians. According to this assumption, the surplus was forcing not a few physicians into other lines of work and was leaving many of the remainder with increasingly precarious incomes from much reduced practices.[5]

The number of physicians at mid-century who could look at this situation dispassionately was doubtless not very large. But some did venture to question whether there was actually a surplus in the regular profession. John K. Mitchell of Philadelphia, in fact, maintained in 1849 that the existing schools were graduating barely half the number of trained medical men needed to keep up with the population, to replace losses of physicians from death or other reasons, and to maintain an average ratio of as high as one physician to 700 persons. Mitchell's fellow-townsman, Robley Dunglison, got an authoritative confirmation of this estimate from the Virginia economist, Professor George Tucker, though Tucker thought that the annual shortage was slightly less than Mitchell did.[6]

Other observers, who endorsed Mitchell and Tucker, went beyond them to demonstrate that the problem was one of distribution as well as supply. It was undeniable that there was a serious surplus of physicians in the larger cities and towns of all geographical areas. For it had long been recognized that cities were natural attractions for physicians and that the largest cities were the most alluring medically. Many, of course, were drawn by the anticipation of a lucrative practice among a well-to-do clientele, and some did indeed realize such a prospect. Some were drawn by social and cultural advantages, and others were attracted by the opportunities for scientific or medical improvement. As Samuel Latham Mitchill noted in 1818, in the city a variety of "infirmaries, hospitals, poorhouses, and dispensaries, afford the means to observe the great variety of accidents and diseases. A great city is in a peculiar manner capable of being rendered a place of instruction."[7]

But if a good many cities had an embarrassment of physicians, it was equally apparent that the thinly populated, newly opening areas of the country had a desperate need for medical personnel. Recognizing this, some antebellum medical editors began to urge the new medical graduates of the day to go west. Such a course would reduce the medical surplus of the cities, and it would virtually eliminate for the graduates the fierce competitive struggles to establish themselves in practice there. As one editor wrote in 1854: "Instead of struggling on through [such] multiplied difficulties, why not strike manfully into the virgin regions of the West, and grow up with society [there], into wealth, usefulness and distinction? . . . Wherever there are human beings, there the advice of the physician is required; and as population increases, so does the odor of his good name. In short, prosperity and usefulness will in most cases be the reward of those who leave the old hive, to act their parts and gather and get gain in the unoccupied localities of Oregon, Nebraska, and Kansas."[8]

Until this advice was widely heeded, of course, many individuals in such areas had to serve as their own doctors. But there were still other problems, besides the imperfect distribution of the profession, which contributed in some measure to keeping physicians from those who needed their services. Some of these problems were especially notice-able in the cities and towns, despite their conspicuous physician sur-pluses. One was the growing factor of poverty among the clientele of nineteenth century urban physicians. If some had an abundance of wealthy and middle class patients, and others found city practice only marginal economically, almost all large-city physicians found them-selves faced with increasing demands upon their time from non-remunerative practice among the poor. While there were obvious limits to what any individual physician could do, doctors were doubtless as motivated as any group by the humanitarian sentiments and projects of the day, and perhaps more so. Some, perhaps most, opened their offices to the poor. And a certain number aided the poor through medical services in almshouses, dispensaries, and hospitals. But, throughout the antebellum period, such institutions in most large cities remained grossly inadequate for the growing swarms of immigrants and other poor. In sum, most cities had enough poor to more than keep their surplus doctors busy, but too few public medical institutions, and too scanty financial means to employ physicians for charity work. As a result, many of the poor failed to get the medical attention they needed and presumably had to resort to inadequate home expedients.

We know a fair amount about the charitable work and other professional activities of the typical nineteenth century physician. But we know relatively little about his non-medical interests and activities, or rather, about their effect upon his medical practice. Carried to an excess, such activities undoubtedly caused some patients to look for different doctors. And repeated absenteeism of the family physician may well have led other sick people to treat themselves.

Cities, of course, offered a wealth of distractions, which could and did draw physicians from their practices. Charles Caldwell advised medical students in the 1830s to take their training in small communities because the expenses, amusements, diversions, and "the incentives to vice of all sorts, are more numerous and powerful in large cities than in small ones."[9] But established physicians themselves often seem to have been no less affected by urban distractions—so much so as to have materially lessened their availability to patients, rich or poor. Politics absorbed a few. Business affairs and speculation in real estate not infrequently took up attention on the side. Service on the governing boards of almshouses, hospitals, schools for the deaf, blind, or orphans, Bible societies, and other charities was time-consuming for some. And the gathering of botanical or zoological specimens, pursuit of agricultural interests, and the organization of medical, scientific, and learned societies took the energies of others. For a single, though doubtless extreme, example of the diversified and thoroughly diverted urban physician, one can point to Samuel Latham Mitchill, a man who, among other things was a busy editor, an active United States Senator, a curious chemist and geologist, an energetic educator, and reputed organizer or member of 49 learned societies. The question has to be asked: how much time was left such a physician to give to his patients?

While such a question can be asked of physicians in New York and other old and settled cities, it is even more pertinent of the profession in the newly established towns and cities of the South and West. Physicians were typically among the founders of these communities, or they settled in them very soon after establishment. In all of them, doctors were diverted at least partially from their functions as medical practitioners to play a variety of leadership roles in the growth and building of the community. Not a few had businesses on the side—banks, stores, interests in railroads. Some speculated in land and wrote propaganda to attract new settlers. Many participated actively in the organization, not only of basic medical institutions, but of museums, lyceums, libraries, colleges, and every sort of intellectual and scientific institution. Some kept meteorological registers; others were pressed into service on state geological surveys. It would be most instructive to learn more accurately the aggregate amount of these outside services or activities; to determine the proportion of physicians who were involved in them; to obtain an informed estimate of the amounts of time lost to medical practice in given cities at given periods of time by the multiple community roles of their physicians.[10]

It seems clear that, as the population grew, both the need and incentive for individual doctors to play outside roles diminished to some extent. Certainly, the number who were pulled away from medicine by scientific interests was never more than a small percentage of the whole. By and large, we have to assume that even in the distracting climate of the nineteenth century, a large proportion of the regular physicians did concentrate on what they were trained to do; they practiced medicine. But whatever importance this fact had for those who were debating the surplus of physicians, it was profoundly irrelevant for many of the people who could not afford the doctors' fees. It also mattered little to those who could not find a doctor when they needed him, to those who were not located within the orbit of a physician's practice, or to those who for various reasons were being led to question the authority and efficacy of the medical profession.

Another of the phenomena which contributed to self-medication during the nineteenth century was the readiness of Americans to pull up their home roots. This propensity, as we know, made mobility into a national characteristic and carried American institutions across a continent. Such mobility was obviously accompanied by its medical hazards, both along the routes of travel and at the points of destination and settlement. There can be no question of the distress and inconvenience which travellers in all periods of history have faced in trying to locate and obtain professional medical assistance in a strange land. Multiply the distressed individual by the hundreds of thousands to gain an idea of the medical problems that Americans separated from their family doctors experienced, often for weeks at a stretch, on the turnpikes to Ohio and Kentucky, on the slow canal barges across New York, up and down the rivers of the great inland basin, by pack train across the vast prairies. Except where there was a physician in the party, travellers who became seriously ill had to wait, with their diseases, until they arrived at some intermediate stop, sometimes after journeying a considerable distance. And medical practitioners at these stops not infrequently accommodated their practices to the needs of these floods of ill travellers, at least those who could pay for care. As an example, when Edward Jarvis arrived at Louisville in 1837, he was quickly advised to set up his office close to the steamboat landing, for "there were frequent calls for a physician on board the boat."[11]

Large numbers of settlers, however, lacked the resources to pay for any kind of comforts along the routes of their travel, let alone medical treatment. And the volume of those travelling in this way, with no economic margin against emergencies, turned out to be far too great for the towns along such routes to cope with. Local physicians, midwives, and others originally did their best to care for the distressed strangers. But it became noticeable in many places, as the westward movement gathered momentum, that the local population gradually hardened to the needs of the migrants. As the clergyman Timothy Flint reported, the "scenes of suffering had become so frequent and familiar, as to have lost their natural tendency to produce sympathy and commiseration."

During the second and third decades of the century, Flint watched these scenes along the Ohio and Mississippi valleys. In Cincinnati, he found large numbers of New Englanders who had "endured great exposure" on the trip West, lying sick and dying in miserable shelters, but friendless and moneyless, and unable to obtain medical help. In New Orleans there were the "multitudes of poor Catholic Irish . . . in crowded apartments [and] unable to help themselves or procure help," who were dying in large numbers of yellow fever, often "unnoticed and unrecorded" by the permanent community. Observers a few years later similarly noted large numbers of poverty-stricken emigrants encamped for months at a time on the edge of St. Louis, "sheltered only by boards temporarily thrown together, . . . badly provided with the necessaries of life, . . . inattentive to the means of preserving health, and negligent of medical advice."[12]

Because of the great distances between stops or towns, travellers often banded together in organized groups that included physicians. But many did not. Such individuals frequently carried a few favorite remedies in their baggage as a precaution against more or less minor indispositions. Some went equipped with fairly elaborate medicine chests which would permit them to cope with almost any emergency themselves. But, while such chests offered some comfort, their owners could count themselves lucky if they did not need to use them.

With or without their medicines, many emigrants could have used the services of physicians before reaching their destinations. Emigrants with severe malarial fevers died on the Indiana prairies in large numbers in 1838 because, although there were a few doctors, there just were not enough of them. Further west, seriously sick emigrants who dragged themselves to one or another of the tiny scattered military posts were out of luck when the detachment and its medical officer were away fighting Indians. And when illness occurred along the trails beyond the outposts of civilization, such as the Overland route through South Pass, there was no possibility of obtaining local care or relief. In 1850, of an estimated 50,000 persons who travelled that route to California, huge numbers suffered from cholera and diarrheas. One observer counted six hundred graves that fall along the south side of the Platte River between the Missouri and Fort Kearney. Along the alternate north side route, however, he found but three graves, though just as many persons had passed along it. He attributed the large difference in mortality chiefly to the fact that the south side had been used mainly by small, largely unorganized groups, while the north side of the river was generally used by the larger organized emigrant parties, many or most of which were accompanied by physicians.[13]

Whatever the medical problems that people encountered along their ways West, they were rarely as serious as the ones they encountered at the sites of their ultimate settlement. Invariably the greatest need for the wisdom of the medical handbook and the few carefully selected remedies came during the first few months or years of settlement. This was the time of "seasoning," a trying period which dampened the optimism of the strongest and took much of the romance out of the western movement. Dismaying quantities of disease and death had, of course, accompanied the "seasoning process" at Plymouth, Jamestown, and many another seventeenth and eighteenth century settle-

41

ment. And they reappeared as inescapable realities at every subsequent forward thrust of the frontier. Where enterprising individuals and families ventured to claim new land out beyond the towns and villages and beyond the physicians, the seasoning process became a particularly direct form of natural selection which took both stamina and luck to survive. Yale President Timothy Dwight observed the operation of the process in his extensive travels around northern New England and western New York around the beginning of the nineteenth century. Like many of his generation, he saw seasoning as partly an environmental matter, one in which an original onslaught of agues, fevers, and vague disabilities was brought on and enhanced by the initial cutting of forests and damming up of streams for mills, but in which such diseases gradually abated as ground was brought under cultivation and civilization was established. But seasoning was also partly a personal matter, the inevitable consequence of diverse physical hardships encountered during the early years of settlement. Dwight specified a number of these conditions, including the necessity of "walking and working a great part of their time in moist ground, the badness of their houses, the poorness of their fare, together with the difficulty of obtaining proper medicines, good nurses, and skillful physicians."[14]

It is likely that travelling medical personnel of one sort or another at least occasionally visited most of the isolated antebellum cabins and farms. For rural and frontier America was kept going by the varied services of its itinerants. Wandering dentists, mesmerists, and healers were thus as conspicuous as the circuit-riding Methodist preachers, the ubiquitous drummers, the enterprising limners and daguerrotype takers. But how many itinerant regular physicians there were is an open question. Small-town doctors did, of course, visit outlying country families. But how often they made such visits, or how far they travelled out of town varied greatly among individuals. Most regular physicians did not find such practice very remunerative. And sometimes they found it difficult to do much for the patient with the limited equipment they carried in their saddlebags. By and large, then, the medical types who visited the more remote habitations tended more often than not to be out-and-out quacks or patent medicine salesmen.

For settlers all over the steadily opening parts of the West, one

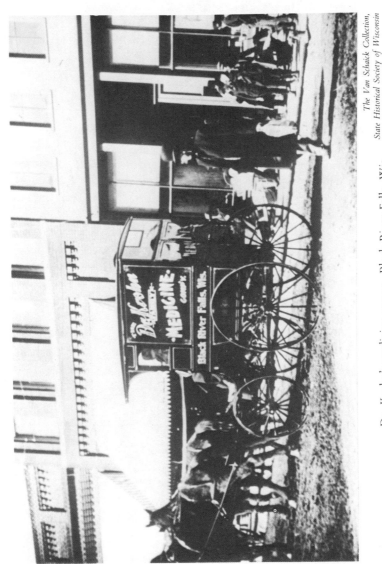

Dr. Krohn's medicine wagon, Black River Falls, Wis.

question remained constant: what to do when serious illness struck between the visits of the doctor, whether he was a regular or an irregular, whether he was competent or a quack? The answers, of course, were much the same as for the emigrant and for the city dweller who could not afford·or did not find regular medical care available. Some let nature take its course or resorted to prayer. Others dosed themselves with whatever medicines were at hand, bound up their wounds, and not infrequently performed surgical operations of one kind or another. Out of primitive necessity, if nothing else, Everyman became his own doctor.

At the same time, some of the accoutrements of man's expanding civilization also facilitated and enhanced the American practice of self-medical care. Prominent among these were the revolutionary advances in transportation and communication, although they had some contradictory effects. On the one hand, the turnpikes and canals, the fast-moving steamboats, and the even swifter railroads helped physicians to spread their practices far more widely than before, while a corps of peripatetic physicians used the new means of travel to move rapidly from one medical school to another hundreds of miles away in successive school terms. On the other hand, rapid transportation and, from the mid-forties, rapid communication in the form of the telegraph, made the tools of the physician—his instruments, drugs, and book knowledge—far more widely attainable than ever before. Book knowledge was a key to the use of the others; and it seemed as if nineteenth century circumstances acted in deliberate concert to improve such knowledge. The development of efficient mail and express systems paralleled as well as expedited the expansion of native publishing houses, the spread of public schools, and the growth of literacy. Doctors of all kinds found it increasingly profitable to write for general audiences. And laymen were increasingly enabled, not only to obtain medical books or tracts for home treatment, but to understand them and use them more or less effectively. The spread of Samuel Thomson's home-oriented botanic system was thus made possible by substantial numbers of at least fairly literate subscribers, as well as by the existence of the means for a rapid distribution of Thomson's books and remedies. And, similarly, the same combination of good transportation and literacy provided a catalyst for the emergence, during the forties and fifties, of new large-volume enterprises catering to personal hygiene and self-medication—popular journals on phrenology and health, inexpensive books and pamphlets on the same subjects from energetic publishers like Fowlers and Wells, with far-flung networks of agents and outlets.

Rapid transportation, of course, also revolutionized the distribution of drugs and medicines from factories through wholesale warehouses and retail outlets—druggists, physicians, or pedlars—to the ultimate consumers. By 1849 a conjunction of the new facilities was making it often fully as easy for the layman as for the physician to obtain drugs and medical equipment rapidly. One enthusiastic Hoosier could hardly say enough good things about the medical benefits of "these happy days of railroads and electric telegraphs. Now, if a man wishes an ounce of morphine or quinine, or a lot of surgical instruments, he [simply] walks to the Telegraph Office . . . and the express will deliver [his order] into his hand, at his own room, in a short time."

Of the mid-century drugs, quinine had quickly become an almost magical word in the United States, especially in the West. On the one hand, physicians found that prescription of this drug was a tremendous boon in their treatment of malarial fevers. At the same time, when individual Americans obtained the drug, as in the form of Sappington's anti-fever pills, they quickly imagined themselves released from much of their need to rely upon doctors. Physicians themselves quickly noted that the use of quinine diminished their roles in the treatment process, and one Midwesterner tried to describe the phenomenon. Ordinarily, he wrote, in periods of great epidemics, "men look to some skilful [sic] physician, and crowd around his door-step or his carriage, besiege his house, and offer up petitions for his services—happy if they can get him to even *promise* them a visit. But here it is the reverse. They look to the medicine alone, as possessing the skill within itself—as though it had intelligence, genius, judgment, learning, all combined."[15]

With such a drug easily available and doctors not always at hand, it was an easy step for not a few nineteenth century Americans to deliberately reject any use of the physician, except perhaps in extreme circumstances. But there were others who rejected drugs as well as physicians. Medical independence had been taking on new dimensions.

For some who had been left to their own medical devices for long years along the frontier, it was undoubtedly simply a matter of a continuing habit. But for many it was a result of their loss of confidence in the medical profession. And for still others, it was the consequence of newly strengthened convictions of the superiority of hygiene over therapy, of preventive medicine over drugging.

The breakdown of the old medical dogmas, of course, was only one of the liberating tendencies of the eighteenth and nineteenth centuries. The medical self-reliance of the individual American was thus reinforced by his fervent pursuit of political suffrage, by his expanding conviction of social egalitarianism, by his rejection of governmental tyranny, and by his skepticism of established religion. And his inclination to be independent of physicians was further encouraged by the romantic revolution in literature and philosophy, with its intense glorification of the individual. Emerson's transcendental celebration of self-reliance went hand in hand with the efforts of health reformers of his generation to give the individual the central responsibility for his own medical well-being. The theme for both was "know thyself." And this was a motto that was readily expandable for that generation to include "improve thyself," "treat thyself," or ultimately, "eliminate the need for medication."

We are unfortunately almost totally ignorant of the various dimensions of domestic medicine at any given time in American history, as well as some of the forces affecting it. We have hardly the slightest idea of its numerical extent, and we know little of its distribution. I would like to see historians make the effort to determine such dimensions, to get at the fundamental quantitative, demographic, and geographic aspects of the subject as well as its qualitative side.

References

[1] James T. Flexner, *Doctors on Horseback: Pioneers of American Medicine* (New York: Dover, 1969).

[2] Samuel Hopkins Adams, "The Vanishing Country Doctor," with sequels, *Ladies Home Journal* 40 (Oct. 1923): 23, 178, 180; (Nov. 1923): 26, 218-220; 41 (Feb. 1924): 31, 149, 150.

[3] Samuel A. Cartwright, "Remarks on Statistical Medicine, contrasting the result of the empirical with the regular practice of Physic, in Natchez," *Western J. Med. Surg.* 2 (1840):

1-21; W.A. Alcott, "Mortality among Children—No. III," *Boston Med. Surg. J.* 51 (1854/55): 260-262; J.V. Prather, "The Causes of Mortality among the Children of St. Louis," *St. Louis Med. Surg. J.* 5 (1847/48): 118-124.

[4] The estimates for the eighteenth century are adapted from the rough figures of Joseph M. Toner, *Contributions to the Annals of Medical Progress and Medical Education in the United States* (Washington: G.P.O., 1874), pp. 105-107. Lemuel Shattuck's Boston census of 1845 identified 566 individuals, classed under 16 different kinds of business, who were "contributors to health." Of that number, 238 were regular or sectarian physicians, which, in a population of 114,000, was one per 479 persons. Lemuel Shattuck, *Report to the Committee of the City Council Appointed to Obtain the Census of Boston for the Year 1845* (Boston: Eastburn, 1846), Appendix Y. See also Charles A. Lee, "Statistics of the Medical Profession in the United States," *Buffalo Med. J.* 10 (1854/55): 203-205.

[5] Charles Caldwell, *Thoughts on the Impolicy of Multiplying Schools of Medicine* (Lexington: Clarke, 1834), pp. 20-23; "Increase of Medical Schools," *Med. Examiner* 2 (1839): 780-781; "New Medical Schools," *The Annalist* 3 (1848/49): 55-56.

[6] John K. Mitchell, "Number of Physicians Required in the United States," *Boston Med. Surg. J.* 42 (1850): 137-139; George Tucker, "On the Proportion of Graduates to the Population," *Buffalo Med. J.* 5 (1849/50): 735-736.

[7] [Samuel L. Mitchill?], "Preface," *Med. Repository* 19 (1818): iv.

[8] Lee, "Statistics of the Medical Profession," pp. 203-205; "Schools of Medicine and Medical Practitioners," *Boston Med. Surg. J.* 50 (1854): 443.

[9] Caldwell, *Thoughts on . . . Schools of Medicine,* pp. 32-34.

[10] A recent study points out that in Paris, Illinois, between 1830 and 1860, physicians, along with lawyers and merchants, "held disproportionately high numbers of leadership roles. Richard S. Alcorn, "Leadership and Stability in Mid-Nineteenth Century America: a Case Study of an Illinois Town," *J. Amer. Hist.* LXI (1974): 697-698.

[11] Edward Jarvis, "[Autobiography, 1803-1873]," manuscript at the Houghton Library, Harvard University, pp. 82 ff.

[12] Timothy Flint, *Recollections of the Last Ten Years* (Boston: Cummings, Hilliard, 1826), pp. 40-41, 311; Prather, "Causes of Mortality . . . of St. Louis," p. 123.

[13] A.B. Shipman, "Professional Matters at the West—Malarious Fever," *Boston Med. Surg. J.* 40 (1849): 69; M.H. Clark, "Mortality on the Platte River," *Boston Med. Surg. J.* 47 (1852/53): 121; "Sad News from the Plains," *Amer. Phrenological J.* 16 (1852): 65.

[14] Timothy Dwight, *Travels in New England and New York,* 4 vols., ed. Barbara Miller Solomon (Cambridge: Harvard University Press, 1969), IV, pp. 77-79.

[15] Shipman, "Professional Matters . . . ," p. 70.

Do-It-Yourself the Sectarian Way*

Ronald L. Numbers

Among the most ardent American champions of home health care were the medical sectarians who arose in the nineteenth century to challenge the heroic therapy of the regulars with their seemingly endless rounds of bleedings, blisterings, and purgings. Over the years a multitude of sects appeared, each offering the long-suffering public a surer, safer, and often cheaper way to health. There were botanics and eclectics, homeopaths and hydropaths, movement-curists and mind-curists, and others too numerous to mention. Despite their many differences, they all shared one trait in common: an enthusiasm for the practice of domestic medicine. Why they felt this way, and how they related their domestic activities to other professional goals, are the questions on which I shall focus. In doing so, I shall look at three of the largest and most influential of the nineteenth century sects: the Thomsonians, the homeopaths, and the hydropaths.

While many nineteenth century domestic medicine books fall under the general heading "botanic," the line between botanic and regular, sectarian and nonsectarian, is often blurred.[1] John Gunn's best-selling *Domestic Medicine,* for example, contains "descriptions of the Medicinal Roots and Herbs of the United States, and how they are to be used in the cure of disease"; yet its tolerance of calomel and bleeding betrays its orthodox origins.[2] Other works on vegetable and Indian medicines were exclusively botanical, but could hardly be called sectarian in the sense of belonging to an exclusive school of medical practice.

The person who turned the root-and-herb tradition into a full-blown medical sect was Samuel Thomson, a New Hampshire farmer who learned much of his botanic medicine at the side of a local female herbalist.[3] Early in his healing career he became convinced that the cause of all disease was cold, and that the only cure was the restoration of the body's natural heat. This he accomplished by steaming, peppering, and puking his patients, with heavy reliance on *lobelia,* an emetic long used by native Americans.[4]

49

The simplicity of his system made it ideal for domestic use. Not one to ignore the commercial possibilities of his discovery, Thomson in 1806 began selling "Family Rights" to his practice, for which he obtained a patent in 1813. For twenty dollars purchasers enrolled in the Friendly Botanic Society and received a sixteen-page instruction booklet, *Family Botanic Medicine*. The section on preparing medicines contained various botanical recipes, but with key ingredients left out. Agents filled in the blanks only after buyers pledged themselves to secrecy "under the penalty of forfeiting their word and honor, and all right to the use of the medicine." By the 1820s Thomson had prepared a more substantial volume entitled *New Guide to Health* (often bound with his autobiography), an edition of which appeared in German for the benefit of recent immigrants.[5]

During the 1820s and 1830s Thomsonian agents fanned out from New England through the southern and western United States urging self-reliant Americans to become their own physicians. Almost everywhere they met with success. By 1840 approximately 100,000 Family Rights had been sold, and Thomson estimated that about three million persons had adopted his system. In states as diverse as Ohio and Mississippi perhaps as many as one-half the citizens were curing themselves the Thomsonian way.[6] And as Daniel Drake observed, the devotees of Thomsonianism were not "limited to the vulgar. Respectable and intelligent mechaniks, legislative and judicial officers, both state and federal barristers, ladies, ministers of the gospel, and even some of the medical profession 'who hold the eel of science by the tail' have become its converts and puffers," he wrote.[7]

The brisk sale of Thomson's *New Guide to Health* encouraged other botanics, including several of Thomson's erstwhile friends, to bring out their own domestic manuals. Elias Smith, once Thomson's general agent, offered a *Medical Pocket-Book, Family Physician, and Sick Man's Guide to Health* as "an extensive improvement" over Thomson's work.[8] Horton Howard, for three and a half years Thomson's agent in Ohio, also broke with the master and published a *Domestic Medicine*.[9] And Morris Mattson, after two frustrating years working with Thomson on a revision of the *New Guide to Health,* finally decided to go it alone with an "improved" guide entitled *The American Vegetable Practice*.[10] Other

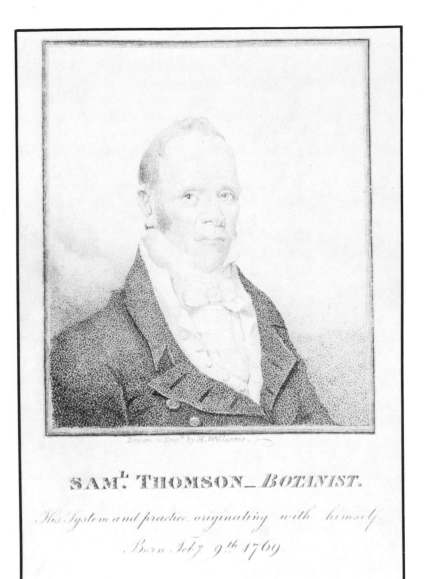

Drawn & Eng^d by H. Williams.

SAM^L. THOMSON _ *BOTANIST*.

His System and practice, originating with himself.

Born Feby 9th 1769.

Portrait of Samuel Thomson.
Frontispiece of his *New Guide to Health*, 1822.

NEW

GUIDE TO HEALTH;

OR,

BOTANIC FAMILY PHYSICIAN.

CONTAINING

A COMPLETE SYSTEM OF PRACTICE,

UPON A PLAN ENTIRELY NEW ;

WITH

A DESCRIPTION OF THE VEGETABLES MADE USE OF, AND DIRECTIONS FOR PREPARING AND ADMINISTERING THEM TO CURE DISEASE.

TO WHICH IS PREFIXED

A NARRATIVE

OF THE

LIFE AND MEDICAL DISCOVERIES

OF THE AUTHOR.

———◆———

BY SAMUEL THOMSON.

———◆———

BOSTON;

PRINTED FOR THE AUTHOR, BY E. G. HOUSE,

No. 18, *Cornhill.*

1822.

Title page of Samuel Thomson's *New Guide to Health,*
1822.

competitors tried to entice potential Thomsonians with offers of books similar in content to the *New Guide* but priced considerably under twenty dollars.[11]

Individuals wishing to practice Thomsonianism at home were not limited to reading books on domestic medicine. They could also subscribe to botanic journals, attend lectures, or correspond directly with Thomsonian practitioners by mail. Among the numerous botanic journals, several were aimed directly at the domestic medicine market. The editor of the Philadelphia-based *Botanic Medical Reformer* declared his intention of making his "sheet a 'HOME PHYSICIAN,'—and to carry to the fireside that knowledge of Medicine which every parent in our land ought to be possessed of."[12] The *Thomsonian Recorder* of Ohio expressed similar sentiments in more picturesque language: "We . . . ardently long to lead our readers away from the rocky cliffs, the miney depths, and the scorching sands of the mineralogical practice, to the fruitful fields, green pastures, and flowery banks of sweetly-gliding streams and grassy fountain sides, to gather roots, and leaves, and blossoms, barks and fruits, for the healing of the nations."[13]

The Thomsonian rallying cry was "Every man his own physician."[14] Unlike many other sectarians, who simply wanted the public to exchange one kind of physician for another, the early Thomsonians seemed genuinely pleased with the prospect of a world without physicians. Given the Jacksonian temper of the times, their slogan had great popular appeal. It reflected both the widespread distrust of elites and the conviction that the head of an American family "should in medicine, as in religion and politics, think and act for himself."[15] It was high time, declared Thomson, for the common man to throw off the oppressive yoke of priests, lawyers, and physicians and assume his rightful place in a truly democratic society.[16]

On a more practical level the Thomsonians argued persuasively that self-medication was safer than being "doctored to death."[17] Again they struck a responsive chord, for Americans in increasing numbers were growing suspicious of the purported benefits of repeated bleedings and calomel dosings. Common people were more likely to place their trust in the healing power of nature and the indigenous remedies that grew around them.[18] They could be sure that their domestically prepared medicines would be "pure, genuine, and unadulterated," unlike those often prepared by apothecaries, or worse yet, their apprentices.[19] Thomsonians frequently commented on the relative safety of their home treatments. "It has been generally remarked," wrote one, "that those families that employ no physicians, in cases of scarlet fever, canker rash, measles, and &c., lose a less number of children, than those who employ them."[20] Another could not recall "a single death from childbed disease" occurring under Thomsonian treatment.[21]

But Thomsonianism offered more than safety. Being your own physician would not only save your life, promised one botanic manual, but your money as well.[22] After the initial outlay of twenty dollars, the Thomsonian family need never worry about exorbitant bills from physicians and apothecaries. This alone, thought Horton Howard, would be sufficient inducement for most people to turn to domestic medicine.[23] The savings often were substantial; one New Hampshire family calculated theirs to be seventy-five dollars a year.[24]

Another unquestioned benefit of home treatment was convenience. "[T]he physician and the cure are always at hand," stressed one Thomsonian. "You have not to wander in the night to a distance, and the patient dying, to seek a doctor, with the agony pressing on your spirits, that your wife, or child, or friend may be dead on your return."[25] And where there were no physicians at all, domestic medicine was not only convenient but necessary. In the western states especially, which sometimes experienced shortages of physicians and apothecaries, self-treatment could be essential.[26] Here the Thomsonians were at a decided advantage, because, as Philip D. Jordan has noted, "most settlers had to supply themselves with drugs, and herbs were easier to secure than chemical mixtures and compounds."[27]

Finally, being your own physician allowed women to avoid the embarrassment of going to male physicians. By adopting Thomsonianism, wrote Horton Howard, women escaped "the necessity of consulting the other sex, with all its attendant indelicacy and mortification."[28] They also won the freedom to practice medicine in a limited way. Joseph Kett has recently argued that Thomsonianism, with its emphasis on the wife and mother as physician, opened medical practice to women "without forcing a confrontation of the sensitive question of whether a woman should ever treat a man other than her husband."[29]

With every person a physician, professional healers were left with few tasks indeed. Samuel Thomson, who opposed even Thomsonian infirmaries and medical schools, would have given them virtually none. If Thomsonian physicians were available, he argued, then people would no longer see the desirability of learning to treat themselves—and perhaps more important, though he did not mention it, they would no longer find it necessary to purchase his Family Rights.[30] Among orthodox Thomsonians, the sole function of physicians was educational. "The physician, instead of dealing out poison," explained one, "would deal out advice to his fellow men to live according to the dictates of nature."[31] He was not to be concerned about the prospect of losing his practice as home treatment increased. Instead, he was to expect to tire of his work after eight or ten years and "be happy to have the people take the burthen of the practice upon themselves."[32]

Not all Thomsonians, however, accepted such a restricted role for trained doctors. Horton Howard recommended resorting to physicians in cases of serious cuts, punctured arteries, broken bones, or unusual or dangerous diseases; and Simon Abbott of Charleston, South Carolina, thought doctors might prove useful for "surgical operations and diseases which rarely occur."[33] This tolerance toward professionals became more common with the opening, over Thomson's adamant opposition, of botanic medical schools in the late 1830s. Naturally those associated with such institutions viewed domestic medicine in a different light from Thomson: home manuals were not to replace the physician but to supplement his efforts.[34] (This was also the opinion of Wooster Beach, founder of the rival eclectic school of medicine and author of two works on home medicine.[35]) Acrimonious debates over such issues as medical education eventually rent the Thomsonians into hostile camps and precipitated the demise of the movement.

As Thomsonian strength began to wane in the 1840s, a new medical sect, homeopathy, was rising to national prominence.[36] Homeopathy was the invention of a regularly educated German physician, Samuel Hahnemann, who had grown dissatisfied with the heroics of orthodox practice. During the last decade of the eighteenth century he began constructing an alternate system based in large part upon the healing power of nature and two fundamental principles, the law of similars and the law of infinitesimals. According to the first law, diseases are cured by medicines having the property of producing in healthy persons symptoms similar to those of the disease. An individual suffering from fever, for example, would be treated with a drug known to increase the pulse rate of a person in health. Hahnemann's second law held that medicines are more efficacious the smaller the dose, even as small as dilutions of up to one-millionth of a gram. Though regular practitioners—or allopaths as Hahnemann called them—ridiculed this theory, many patients flourished under homeopathic treatment and they seldom suffered.

Following its appearance in this country in 1825, homeopathy rapidly grew into a major medical sect. By the outbreak of the Civil War there were nearly 2,500 homeopathic physicians, concentrated largely in New England, New York, Pennsylvania, and the Midwest, and hundreds of thousands of devoted followers.[37] Homeopathy's appeal is not difficult to understand. Instead of the bleedings and purgings of the regulars, or the equally rigorous therapy of the Thomsonians, the homeopaths offered pleasant-tasting pills that produced no discomforting side effects. Such medication was particularly suitable for babies and small children. As the orthodox Oliver Wendell Holmes observed, homeopathy "does not offend the palate, and so spares the nursery those scenes of single combat in which infants were wont to yield at length to the pressure of the spoon and the imminence of asphyxia."[38] Perhaps because of its suitability for children, homeopathy won the support of large numbers of American women, who constituted approximately two-thirds of its patrons and who were among its most active propagators. "Many a woman, armed with her little stock of remedies, has converted an entire community," proudly reported the American Institute of Homeopathy.[39]

Central to the home practice of homeopathy was the "domestic kit," which consisted of a case of infinitesimal medicines and a guide. Scores if not hundreds of these were available during the nineteenth century in a variety of combinations ranging from small pocket cases with tiny guides to large family chests with thick volumes. Often the books appeared in foreign languages as well as in English, and occasionally they included homeopathic treatments for domestic animals.[40]

The first such kit came from the hands of Constantine Hering, a Leipzig-educated physician who settled in Pennsylvania in the early 1830s and who did as much as any man to promote the cause of homeopathy in America. In 1835 he published the first part of *The Homoeopathist, or Domestic Physician,* and three years later he completed the second part. These he sold, together with a small mahogany box of medicines, for five dollars (four dollars for the German edition). The box contained small numbered vials filled with "infinitesimal pills," the numbers on the vials corresponding to the numbered remedies in the book. Self-treatment, once a diagnosis was made, was thus reduced simply to taking a No. 8 or a No. 17 pill, or whatever the manual recommended.[41]

Since most homeopaths were, like Hahnemann and Hering, trained physicians, they understandably did not share the Thomsonian enthusiasm for making every man a physician. Besides, many were recent immigrants from Germany, uninfected by Jacksonian democracy. They envisioned only a limited role for domestic practice. Hering, for example, wrote his book not to replace the physician but to assist families in treating minor complaints and to provide medical advice for students, travellers, mariners, and "those living in remote parts of the country." Like virtually all his homeopathic colleagues, he urged his readers to seek qualified medical assistance in serious cases.[42]

Several homeopathic domestic guides pointedly discouraged self-treatment. One warned that since even physicians could not safely treat themselves, ordinary persons should not think they could. George E. Shipman's popular *Homoeopathic Family Guide* cautioned that "No *very* sensible person will ever attempt to treat himself or his family, who can obtain the advice of a well-qualified physician. If those fail too often, who make the study of disease and their remedies the sole business of their lives," wrote Shipman, "what success can they expect, who know little or nothing of either?"[43]

But regardless of their reservations about home treatment, homeopaths were well aware that the domestic kits were one of their most effective weapons in winning converts from the allopaths. The domestic guides, especially in the early days, were seen as "missionaries of truth" preparing the way for the arrival of homeopathic physicians. Thus most homeopaths viewed domestic manuals not as competitors, but "as necessary allies in the great work of reforming the medical state of the world."[44] Even allopaths did not dispute their effectiveness. Many an "impecunious practitioner" has failed to get a case, complained one regular, because of "Dr. Humphreys' book and box that preceded him in the domestic corner."[45]

The homeopaths also derived encouragement from the knowledge that their practice was relatively harmless—certainly safer than "the Old System of Physic," "whose gentlest weapons are lancets and cathartics." Even if the patient took the wrong medicine, there was no need for alarm, wrote Hering, "for Homoeopathic medicine is so prepared that it will help, when it is the right one, but it will not injure should a mistake occur." The very worst possibility would be a slight delay in the healing process.[46] Readers of one manual were assured that "No life was ever lost by homoeopathic medicine used carelessly, or otherwise," a point conceded by sarcastic allopaths. Homeopathy, wrote Dr. Holmes, "gives the ignorant, who have such an inveterate itch for dabbling in physic, a book and a doll's medicine chest, and lets them play doctors and doctresses without fear of having to call in the coroner."[47]

Domestic homeopathy was not, however, without its difficulties, and its advocates were continually devising new ways of facilitating its practice. As in all forms of home treatment, making a correct diagnosis was probably the greatest challenge to the uninitiated, especially if there were a multitude of symptoms. To assist the bewildered domestic practitioner, one enterprising homeopath invented an elaborate but foolproof diagnostic system composed of a small book listing 2,467 symptoms and a pasteboard box filled with 2,467 numbered slips of paper, one per symptom. On each slip appeared the names of 127 remedies, with assigned weights from one to four. Users were instructed to select the slips corresponding to each of their symptoms, line them up in a row, identify the remedies found on every slip, add the weights for each remedy, and take the one with the highest total. In case of a tie, users were to "select from among the symptoms whichever one seems the most peculiar, or important, and take the rating of the remedies in question there given, as your indication for choice."[48]

Frederick Humphreys, mentioned earlier, discovered another method of simplifying home medication. A sometime professor in the Homeopathic Medical College of Pennsylvania, Humphreys broke with Hahnemann's rule of administering only one medicine at a time and instead recommended combinations of medicines for specific diseases, manufactured by his own Specific Homeopathic Medicine Company. Although some uncharitable colleagues called his invention "Homeopathic quackery," lay homeopaths seem to have thought otherwise. The sale of his two domestic guides, a large one to accompany his more expensive kits and a smaller one for his cheaper cases, was truly phenomenal. By the early 1890s 15,000,000 copies of the latter work had appeared in five languages, 12,000,000 of which had been distributed in the United States. In one year alone he printed 3,000,000 copies.[49]

Despite the safety and popularity of these domestic kits and their acknowledged role in diffusing the principles of homeopathy, a few homeopaths questioned what they saw as an over-emphasis on home medical care. John Ellis of Cleveland thought that books on preventive medicine were far more important "than any work on domestic medicine can possibly be," and claimed that his own *Family Homoeopathy* was written primarily to direct attention to his earlier but often ignored work on *The Avoidable Causes of Disease*.[50] *The Family Journal of Homoeopathy,* published by a group of St. Louis physicians, went even further in condemning "domestic practice of every description." "[W]e would prefer a good Allopath to prescribe for us than an ignorant or mongrel Homoeopath," the editors declared.[51]

As the century progressed and homeopathy came to occupy a secure place in American medicine, homeopaths began directing their attention less to the general public and more toward their own profession.[52] The writings of Charles J. Hempel, who authored a *Homoeopathic Domestic Physician* in 1846, reflect this change. After issuing two editions of his home guide, he became increasingly pessimistic about the value of domestic practice and decided, instead of preparing a third edition, to publish a volume on *Homoeopathic Theory and Practice,* "designed both for the public and for students and practitioners."[53]

The domestic guides that continued to appear during the latter part of the century tended to be somewhat less comprehensive than their predecessors and to focus instead on emergency care and minor diseases. There is no longer any need to provide every person with the "knowledge of a physician," wrote one homeopath in 1887, "for the doctor himself is at hand in every village and hamlet of the land, ready at the first summons to give advice and assistance far more valuable than that of any book."[54] This situation did not last long, however, if in fact it ever existed. Within a few decades homeopathy was fast fading from sight, and the question of homeopathic domestic practice had become moot.

To escape the most obvious pitfalls of allopathic practice, the Thomsonians had turned to botanic remedies and the homeopaths to their infinitesimal pills. A third sect, hydropathy, rejected drugs of every variety, whether botanic or mineral, in large or small doses. The hydropaths placed their trust solely in natural cures like fresh air, sunshine, exercise, proper (often vegetarian) diet, and, above all, water, which they used in every conceivable way.[55]

Hydropathy was a mélange of water treatments devised by a Silesian peasant, Vincent Priessnitz, to heal his wounds after accidentally being run over by a wagon. His therapy proved so successful that he opened his home in Graefenberg as a "water cure" and invited his ailing neighbors to submit their bodies to a bewildering variety of baths, packs, and wet bandages. When news of his methods reached the United States in the mid-1840s, it touched off a water-cure craze that continued unabated until the outbreak of the Civil War. Two regularly educated physicians, Joel Shew and Russell T. Trall, opened the first American water-cure establishments in New York City about 1843. A couple of years later Mary Gove (Nichols), an experienced woman health reformer, opened still a third water cure in the city. It was primarily these three pioneers—Shew, Trall, and Nichols—who introduced Americans to the new water system.

Among them they wrote perhaps a dozen volumes for domestic

use. Throughout their writings run many of the themes commonly found in sectarian guides: the economy and absolute safety of their practice, the importance of prevention, and the advantages of self-reliance. On the question of making every man a physician, they fell somewhere between the early radical Thomsonians and the more moderate homeopaths. Since all three writers operated commercial water cures, they could hardly deny the value of professional care; yet they realized that relatively few people had access to such establishments or to hydropathic physicians, of which there were never many.[56]

In theory they saw little justification for limiting self-practice. The water treatments themselves were harmless, with the possible exception of the powerful douche, which one author warned should be used "with great caution, and always under the direction of an experienced hydropathic physician."[57] In Shew's opinion, hydropathy was "destined, not only to make the members of communities their own physicians for the most part, but to mitigate, in an unprecedented manner, the extent, the pains, and the perils of disease." The only time when professional assistance might be necessary was in the event of a serious injury, like a skull fracture.[58] Trall's attitude was basically the same. When the people become familiar with the principles of hydropathy and the laws of life and health, he predicted, "they will well-nigh emancipate themselves from all need of doctors of any sort." He thought home practitioners could successfully treat functional problems, which he estimated to be 99 percent of all ailments, but that they would probably need the skill of a trained surgeon for "mechanical injuries, displacements of parts, organic lesions, etc."[59]

Mrs. Nichols, the only nonphysician of the three, looked forward expectantly to the day when the spread of hydropathy would make physicians obsolete. Since a water-cure family seldom needed a physician more than once, she foresaw the end of medical practice outside the home. "Mothers learn to not only cure the disease of their families, but, what is more important, to keep them in health," she wrote in 1849. "The only way a Water Cure physician can live, is by constantly getting new patients, as the old ones are too thoroughly cured, and too well informed, to require further advice. This is a striking advantage to Water Cure patients, if not to Water Cure physicians."[60]

Like Thomsonians, hydropaths placed special emphasis on the role of women as providers and consumers of health care. In an age of few female doctors, roughly one-fifth of professional hydropaths were women.[61] Many water-curists of both sexes actively participated in the antebellum feminist movement, particularly as it related to freeing women from their "clothes-prisons" and from the dominance of male physicians. As part of their effort to effect the latter goal, they prepared domestic manuals instructing women on the care of their own bodies, as well as on the care of their families.[62]

One of the most successful means of popularizing all facets of hydropathy was the *Water-Cure Journal,* first published by Shew in 1845 and later edited by Trall. Beginning with the third volume, Shew promised to include considerable advice on domestic treatment, "thus enabling persons who cannot visit a hydropathic establishment, to prescribe for themselves." Those desiring more specific counsel than that printed in the journal were invited to correspond with the editor directly, on condition that they send a fee in advance.[63] Because of the scarcity of hydropathic physicians, several practitioners, including Mrs. Nichols, resorted to this semi-domestic device.

Numerous letters from *Journal* readers demonstrate the great popularity of domestic hydropathy and the eagerness of home practitioners to relate their experiences. One elderly man from Missouri vividly described his treatment for fever in the following letter to the publishers:

> . . . I put the patient in a hogshead that I keep for bathing. I have him go entirely under water, head and all, for three or four times, keeping his head under each time as long as he can conveniently hold his breath; then let him dabble in it up to the chin until the heat is reduced to the normal temperature, and the patient feels comfortable . . . . When I have no convenience for bathing, and, in fact, sometimes, as a matter of preference, I pour water on the patient's head, instead of bathing; and, surprising as it may seem, this always has the same effect that bathing has . . . . I have the patient lie with the head over the edge or side of the bed, so that the water will not wet the bedding. I then get a bucket of the coldest water . . . . the cure is completed in a few minutes, and it is a permanent cure, and a cure that all persons can perform at home without any inconvenience.[64]

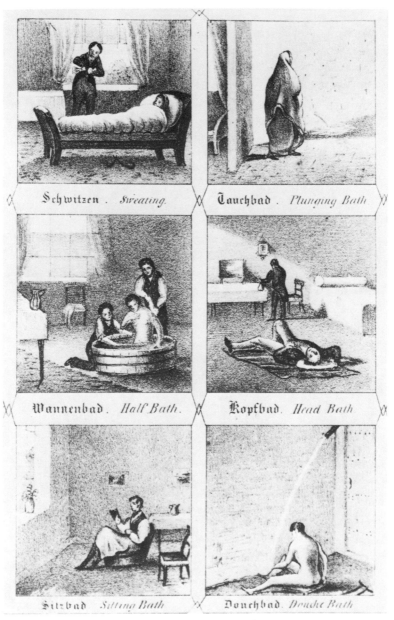

Common water cure procedures.
From *Water-Cure for Ladies,* by Mrs. M. L. Shew, 1844.

Besides the *Water-Cure Journal* there were a number of lesser hydropathic magazines vying for the public's attention. One of the best of these was the *Laws of Life,* published in Dansville, New York, at Our Home on the Hillside, an unusually successful water cure operated by James Caleb Jackson and a woman associate.[65] During the waning years of the water-cure movement Jackson turned out a steady stream of works on home hydropathy, including a volume on the treatment of sexual disorders (a favorite topic of many health reformers) and a comprehensive and widely read book on *How to Treat the Sick without Medicine.*[66]

In one sense Jackson's most influential work on domestic medicine may have been a short essay on curing diphtheria with water, which appeared in an upstate New York newspaper during a diphtheria epidemic in the winter of 1862–63. Somehow this paper reached Battle Creek, Michigan, and fell into the hands of Ellen G. White, prophetess of the Seventh-day Adventist church and mother of two boys suffering from sore throats and high fevers. Hopefully she applied the recommended fomentations and met "with perfect success."[67] Several months later, during one of her frequent religious trances, God directed her to lead her Adventist followers into the hydropathic fold. As a result of her labors, in 1866 the Adventists opened their own water cure in Battle Creek and began publishing a hydropathic journal called *The Health Reformer,* which featured answers to questions on home water treatments.[68]

Even more important for the future of domestic hydropathy was Mrs. White's influence on her protégé John Harvey Kellogg (of corn-flake fame), whom she and her husband assisted with obtaining both hydropathic and regular medical degrees. Kellogg in turn became the most prolific writer on domestic hydropathy—or hydrotherapy as it came to be called—during the late nineteenth and early twentieth centuries, authoring such works as *The Household Manual of Domestic Hygiene, Ladies' Guide in Health and Disease, The Household Monitor of Health,* and *The Home Hand-Book of Domestic Hygiene and Rational Medicine,* which sold nearly a hundred thousand copies during its first twenty-five years.[69] Kellogg was the last of the major writers of domestic hydropathic guides, but well into the twentieth century there appeared an occasional home manual advocating hydrotherapy as the safest of all therapies.[70] These books, however, were largely devoid of sectarian spirit and probably differed more from Shew's and Trall's early handbooks than from the orthodox guides of the day.

This brief look at sectarian domestic medicine reveals something of the extent to which home health care permeated American society during the nineteenth century. For literally millions of Americans, the sectarian domestic guides served as primary care physicians. While it is true that much of the sectarian literature simply reflected orthodox concerns with cost, convenience, and accessibility of doctors, in many respects the sectarian tradition was unique: in its exploitation of the therapeutic weaknesses of regular medicine, in its more ready acceptance of domestic medicine as a substitute for professional health care, and in its missionary zeal. In view of the effectiveness of domestic medicine in making and holding sectarian converts, it is no exaggeration to say that home health care was the foundation upon which the American medical sects were built.

References

*I wish to thank Blanche L. Singer, of the Middleton Medical Library, University of Wisconsin, and Janet Schulze Numbers for their assistance in the preparation of this paper.

[1] See Alex Berman, "The Impact of the Nineteenth Century Botanico-Medical Movement on American Pharmacy and Medicine" (unpublished Ph.D. dissertation, University of Wisconsin, 1954), pp. 92–93.

[2] John Gunn, *Gunn's Domestic Medicine, or Poor Man's Friend* 1st rev. ed. (Philadelphia: G.V. Raymond, 1839). On the popularity of Gunn's book, see Madge E. Pickard and R. Carlyle Buley, *The Midwest Pioneer: His Ills, Cures, and Doctors* (New York: Henry Schuman, 1946), p. 93.

[3] Berman's unpublished dissertation remains the most thorough treatment of Thomsonianism; but see also Alex Berman, "The Thomsonian Movement and Its Relation to American Pharmacy and Medicine," *Bulletin of the History of Medicine* XXV (Sept.-Oct. 1951): 405–428; (Nov.-Dec. 1951): 519–538; Pickard and Buley, *The Midwest Pioneer,* Chap. 4, pp. 167–198; Joseph F. Kett, *The Formation of the American Medical Profession: The Role of Institutions, 1780–1860* (New Haven: Yale University Press, 1968), Chap. 4, pp. 97–131; and James Harvey Young, *The Toadstool Millionaires: A Social History of Patent Medicines in America before Federal Regulation* (Princeton: Princeton University Press, 1961), Chap. 4, pp. 44–57.

4 Samuel Thomson, *New Guide to Health; or, Botanic Family Physician* 2nd ed. (Boston: For the author, 1825), Part 1, pp. 42–45.

5 *Ibid.*, Part 2, p. 4; Samuel Thomson, *Family Botanic Medicine* (Boston: T.G. Bangs, 1819).

6 Berman, "The Impact of the Nineteenth Century Botanico-Medical Movement . . . ," pp. 150–152.

7 Daniel Drake, "The People's Doctors," *Western Journal of the Medical and Physical Sciences* (1829): 407, quoted *ibid.*, pp. 42–43.

8 Elias Smith, *The Medical Pocket-Book, Family Physician, and Sick Man's Guide to Health* (Boston: Henry Bowen, 1822), p. viii. Four years later Smith published *The American Physician, and Family Assistant* (Boston: E. Bellamy, 1826) as an improvement over his own *Medical Pocket-Book.*

9 Horton Howard, *Howard's Domestic Medicine* New Enlarged ed. (Philadelphia: Duane Rulison, 1866).

10 Morris Mattson, *The American Vegetable Practice, or A New and Improved Guide to Health Designed for the Use of Families* (Boston: Daniel L. Hale, 1841).

11 See, for example, Reuben Chambers, *The Thomsonian Practice of Medicine* (Bethania, Penn., 1842).

12 Editorial, *Botanic Medical Reformer and Home Physician* I (May 7, 1840): 9–10.

13 Preface to Vol. II, *Thomsonian Recorder* (1833): p. v.

14 See Thomson, *New Guide to Health,* Part 1, p. 10. This motto, or variations of it, appears in numerous botanic works on domestic medicine.

15 William Procter, Jr., *American Journal of Pharmacy* XXVI (1854): 570, quoted in Berman, "The Impact of the Nineteenth Century Botanico-Medical Movement . . . ," pp. 40–41.

16 Thomson, *New Guide to Health,* Part 2, p. 5.

17 Howard, *Howard's Domestic Medicine,* p. 30.

18 See, for example, Elisha Smith, *The Botanic Physician; Being a Compendium of the Practice of Physic, upon Botanical Principles* (New York: Murphy and Bingham, 1830), p. vi.

19 L. Sperry, *The Botanic Family Physician, or The Secret of Curing Diseases with Vegetable Proportions* (Cornwall, Vt.: By the author, 1843), p. 5.

20 Benjamin Colby, *A Guide to Health: Being an Exposition of the Principles of the Thomsonian System of Practice* (Nashua, N.H.: Charles T. Gill, 1844), p. x.

21 J.W. Comfort, *Thomsonian Practice of Midwifery* (Philadelphia: Aaron Comfort, 1845), p. iii.

22 F.K. Robertson and Silas Wilcox, *The Book of Health, or Thomsonian Theory and Practice of Medicine* (Bennington, Vt.: J.I.C. & A.S.C. Cook, 1843), p. 5.

23 Howard, *Howard's Domestic Medicine,* p. 427.

24 Colby, *A Guide to Health,* p. x.

25 Simon Abbott, *The Southern Botanic Physician* (Charleston: For the author, 1844), p. ix.

[26] P.E. Sanborn urged husbands emigrating West to learn the art of midwifery, since "many females suffer and die in some parts of the West, for want of medical skill and attention." Sanborn, *The Sick Man's Friend* (Taunton, Mass.: By the author, 1835), p. 237.

[27] Philip D. Jordan, "The Eclectic of St. Clairsville," *Ohio State Archaeological and Historical Quarterly* LVI (October 1947): 391.

[28] Howard, *Howard's Domestic Medicine,* p. 286.

[29] Kett, *The Formation of the American Medical Profession,* p. 119.

[30] Samuel Thomson, Editorial, *Thomsonian Manual* I (August 15, 1836): 153.

[31] Colby, *A Guide to Health,* p. viii.

[32] Robertson and Wilcox, *The Book of Health . . . ,* p. 19.

[33] Howard, *Howard's Domestic Medicine,* pp. 30–32; Abbott, *The Southern Botanic Physician,* p. v.

[34] See, for example, Wm. H. Cook, *Woman's Hand-Book of Health: A Guide for the Wife, Mother and Nurse* 5th ed. (Cincinnati: Wm. H. Cook, 1871). Cook was professor of botany, therapeutics, and materia medica in the Physio-Medical Institute.

[35] Wooster Beach, *The American Practice Condensed, or the Family Physician* 10th ed. (New York: James McAlister, 1847), p. xv. Beach also published *The Family Physician; or The Reformed System of Medicine on Vegetable or Botanical Principles* (New York: By the author, 1842.)

[36] On homeopathy in America, see Martin Kaufman, *Homeopathy in America: The Rise and Fall of a Medical Heresy* (Baltimore: Johns Hopkins Press, 1971); Harris L. Coulter, *Divided Legacy: A History of the Schism in Medical Thought* (Washington, D.C.: McGrath Publishing Co., 1973), Vol. 3; and Kett, *The Formation of the American Medical Profession,* Chap. 5, pp. 132–164.

[37] Coulter, *Divided Legacy,* Vol. 3, pp. 101–110.

[38] Oliver Wendell Holmes, "Some More Recent Views on Homoeopathy," *Atlantic Monthly* (December 1857): 187, quoted *ibid.,* p. 114.

[39] *Ibid.,* pp. 114–116.

[40] See, for example, C.S. and George E. Halsey, *Halsey's Homoeopathic Guide: For Families, Travelers, Missionaries, Pioneers, Miners, Farmers, Stock Raisers, Horse Owners, Dog Fanciers, Poultry Keepers* (Chicago: C.S. and George E. Halsey, 1885). Domestic manuals appear with great frequency in Thomas Lindsley Bradford, *Homoeopathic Bibliography of the United States, from the Year 1825 to the Year 1891, Inclusive* (Philadelphia: Boericke and Tafel, 1892).

[41] C. Hering, *The Homoeopathist, or Domestic Physician* Two parts (Philadelphia: J.G. Wesselhoeft, 1835, 1838); Coulter, *Divided Legacy,* Vol. 3, pp. 101-102; Bradford, *Homoeopathic Bibliography . . . ,* p. 145.

[42] Hering, *The Homoeopathist . . . ,* Part 1, pp. 2-3; Part 2, p. 241.

[43] Morton M. Eaton, *Eaton's Domestic Practice for Parents and Nurses* (Cincinnati: M.M. Eaton, Jr., and Co., 1882), p. 77; George E. Shipman, *The Homoeopathic Family Guide* 2nd ed. (Chicago: C.S. Halsey, 1865), p. ix.

[44] J.H. Pulte, *Homeopathic Domestic Physician; Containing the Treatment of Diseases, with Popular*

Explanations on Anatomy, Physiology, Hygiene, and Hydropathy (Cincinnati: H.W. Derby and Co., 1850), pp. iv–v. See also E.H. Ruddock, *The Stepping-Stone to Homoeopathy and Health,* ed. Wm. Boericke. New Am. ed. (Philadelphia: Hahnemann Publishing House, 1890), p. 10.

45Quoted in Coulter, *Divided Legacy,* Vol. 3, p. 117.

46Egbert Guernsey, *The Gentleman's Hand-Book of Homoeopathy; Especially for Travelers, and for Domestic Practice* (Boston: Otis Clapp, 1855), p. iv; Hering, *The Homoeopathist . . . ,* Part 1, p. 7; John Epps, *Domestic Homoeopathy,* ed. George W. Cook. 4th Am. ed. (Boston: Otis Clapp, 1849), p. 8.

47E.R. Ellis, *Homoeopathic Family Guide and Information for the People* 2nd ed. (Detroit: By the author, 1882), p. ii; Holmes, "Some More Recent Views on Homoeopathy," p. 187, quoted in Coulter, *Divided Legacy,* Vol. 3, p. 116.

48Bradford, *Homoeopathic Bibliography . . . ,* pp. 99–100.

49Frederick Humphreys, *Manual of Specific Homoeopathy* (New York: Humphreys' Specific Homoeopathic Medicine Company, 1869); *Humphreys' Homeopathic Mentor or Family Adviser* (New York: Humphreys' Specific Homeopathic Medicine Company, 1876); Bradford, *Homoeopathic Bibliography . . . ,* p. 167. The reference to "Homoeopathic quackery" is from J.S. Douglas, *Practical Homoeopathy for the People* 15th ed. (Milwaukee: Lewis Sherman, 1894), p. iii.

50John Ellis, *Personal Experience of a Physician* (Philadelphia: Hahnemann Publishing House, 1892), pp. 85–87.

51"Domestic Practice.—No. 2, " *Family Journal of Homoeopathy* I (July 1854): 105. See also Guernsey's reply to the criticisms against domestic practice; Guernsey, *The Gentleman's Hand-Book of Homoeopathy,* p. iv.

52"Progress of Homeopathy," *Homoeopathic Sun* I (September 1868): 12.

53Charles J. Hempel, *The Homoeopathic Domestic Physician* (New York: Wm. Radde, 1846); Hempel and Jacob Beakley, *Homoeopathic Theory and Practice* 4th ed. (New York: William Radde, 1868), p. iii.

54Henry G. Hanchett, *The Elements of Modern Domestic Medicine* (New York: Charles T. Hurlburt, 1887), p. 3.

55On hydropathy in America, see Harry B. Weiss and Howard R. Kemble, *The Great American Water-Cure Craze: A History of Hydropathy in the United States* (Trenton, N.J.: Past Times Press, 1967); and Marshall Scott Legan, "Hydropathy in America: A Nineteenth Century Panacea," *Bulletin of the History of Medicine* XLV (May-June 1971): 267–280.

56Weiss and Kemble, *The Great American Water-Cure Craze,* (p. 44) were able to identify only 241 American hydropathic physicians.

57David A. Harsha, *The Principles of Hydropathy, or the Invalid's Guide to Health and Happiness* (Albany, N.Y.: E.H. Pease & Co., 1852), p. 41.

58Joel Shew, *The Hydropathic Family Physician* (New York: Fowler and Wells, 1854), p. iii; Shew, *The Water-Cure Manual: A Popular Work* (New York: Fowlers and Wells, 1855), p. 132. Shew's *Hand-Book of Hydropathy* (New York: Wiley & Putnam, 1844), was probably the first American domestic guide to hydropathy.

[59] R.T. Trall, American preface to William Horsell, *Hydropathy for the People* (New York: Fowlers and Wells, 1855), p. iii; Trall, *The Hydropathic Encyclopedia: A System of Hydropathy and Hygiene* (New York: Fowler and Wells, 1851), I, p. 295.

[60] Mary S. Gove Nichols, *Experience in Water-Cure: A Familiar Exposition of the Principles and Results of Water Treatment, in the Cure of Acute and Chronic Diseases* (New York: Fowlers and Wells, 1852), p. 10.

[61] Weiss and Kemble, *The Great American Water-Cure Craze,* p. 44.

[62] See, for example, Mary S. Gove, *Lectures to Women on Anatomy and Physiology, with an Appendix on Water Cure* (New York: Harper and Brothers, 1846); and M. Augusta Fairchild, *How to Be Well, or Common-Sense Medical Hygiene* (New York: Fowler & Wells, 1880).

[63] *Water-Cure Journal* II (November 1, 1846): 168; *ibid.* VI (1848): 138. An example of how domestic practice supplemented the use of water-cure establishments is found in the diary of Mrs. Angeline Stevens Andrews, 1863-64 (C. Burton Clark Collection, Heritage Room, Loma Linda University Library).

[64] Abraham Millar to Fowlers and Wells, November 30, 1850, quoted in Trall, *Hydropathic Encyclopedia,* II, pp. 81-82.

[65] According to the editor, Harriet N. Austin, one of the purposes of the journal was to give "directions for the rational and successful treatment of all [disease]"; *Laws of Life* VIII (August, 1865): 127.

[66] James C. Jackson, *The Sexual Organism, and Its Healthful Management* (Boston: B. Leverett Emerson, 1861); Jackson, *How to Treat the Sick without Medicine* 10th ed. (Dansville, New York: Austin, Jackson & Co., 1880). See also Jackson, *Consumption: How to Prevent It, and How to Cure It* (Boston: B. Leverett Emerson, 1862); and Jackson, *Diptheria* [*sic*]: *Its Causes, Treatment and Cure* (Dansville, N.Y.: Austin, Jackson and Co., 1868).

[67] *Advent Review and Sabbath Herald* XXI (February 17, 1863): 89.

[68] H.S. Lay, "To the Reader," *Health Reformer* I (August 1866): 8; "Items for the Month," *ibid.* I (January 1867): 96. On Ellen White and Adventist health reform, see Ronald L. Numbers, *Prophetess of Health: A Study of Ellen G. White* (New York: Harper & Row, 1976).

[69] [John Harvey Kellogg], *The Household Manual of Domestic Hygiene, Foods and Drinks, Common Diseases, Accidents and Emergencies, and Useful Hints and Recipes* (Battle Creek: Modern Medicine Publishing Co., 1893); Kellogg, *Ladies' Guide in Health and Disease* (Battle Creek: Modern Medicine Publishing Co., 1893); Kellogg, *The Household Monitor of Health* (Battle Creek: Good Health Publishing Co., 1891); Kellogg, *The Home Hand-Book of Domestic Hygiene and Rational Medicine* Rev. ed. (Battle Creek: Modern Medicine Publishing Co., 1906). The last work was first published in 1880. Kellogg's older half-brother Merritt also wrote domestic manuals; see [M.G. Kellogg], *The Hygienic Family Physician: A Complete Guide for the Preservation of Health, and the Treatment of the Sick without Medicine* (Battle Creek: Health Reformer, 1874); and M.G. Kellogg, *The Bath: Its Use and Application* (Battle Creek: Health Reformer, 1873).

[70] See, for example, Newton Evans, Percy T. Magan, and George Thomason (eds.), *The Home Physician and Guide to Health* (Mountain View, California: Pacific Press, 1923): and Hubert O. Swartout, *Guide to Health* (Mountain View, California: Pacific Press, 1938).

Nineteenth Century Health Reform and Women: A Program of Self-Help*

Regina Markell Morantz

Domestic medicine enjoys a long and distinguished history. The popularity in colonial America of several practical guides to good health attests to the colonists' interest in self-dosing. In the years after 1830, however, concern with personal health and hygiene intensified. The social historian must come to terms with a new phenomenon: the emergence of a coherent and articulate campaign to save the nation by combating the ill-health of its citizenry. A health reform movement, exhibiting all the characteristics of a full-fledged moral crusade, was born.

There are many reasons why good health emerged as a pressing issue for Jacksonian Americans. The health crusade coincided with several better known antebellum reform causes, and the large majority of health reformers—men and women alike—supported other meliorist programs like abolitionism and women's rights. Itinerant abolitionist speakers lodged in health reform boarding houses, and a number of early feminists followed some form of the Graham diet. Nor was this occurrence merely fortuitous. Health reform constituted part of a larger cultural response to the pressures and strains of a modernizing nation. It shared with other reforms a particular angle of vision, a distinctive way of viewing the world.

The following will attempt neither to describe the movement in detail, nor to account definitively for its emergence. On the contrary, the focus of this study will be less ambitious: to explore the connection between health reform and one specific group: middle class American women. Several of the most outspoken of the health crusaders were female, and women swelled the rank and file of the new movement. Such participation took place in a period when many women were experiencing profound and unsettling changes in their lives. What did health reform offer these women, and how did their response affect the

73

character of the movement? The answers to these and similar questions should do more than tell us something about the lives of women in this period, they should illuminate yet another aspect of the reformist mind.

"The time is passing—" warned Ann Preston in her 1851 graduate medical thesis on "General Diagnosis," "when . . . the licensed graduate whose lancet is sprung for every head-ache and *heart-ache* that he may meet can obtain public confidence." Preston, soon to become dean of her alma mater, the newly established Female Medical College of Pennsylvania, voiced what was by 1851 a lively public issue. Her fellow classmate, Angenette A. Hunt, echoed Preston's admonition when she observed in her own thesis that the present public criticism of the medical profession was well deserved: "The merit of the Physician," she declared vehemently, "is not now estimated by the quantity of medicines he prescribes, but by the effect produced, and the public throat is rebelling against swallowing nauseous drugs for the pleasure and profit of the doctors." What is more, continued Hunt, "public opinion is beginning to prove that there is a female side to *this subject,* as well as most others." Woman had natural abilities which made her peculiarly fitted for health care. With proper education, woman could exercise her talents and move in the process to a higher sphere, "one not bounded," Hunt added, "by the kitchen and the nursery."[1]

By mid-century criticism of established medical practice had reached astonishing proportions; doctors had good reason to feel on the defensive. "The practice, or so-called *science* of medicine, has been little else than one of experiment," observed Mrs. Marie Louise Shew in a scathing indictment. Standard medical therapeutics, she claimed, had hitherto been characterized by "uncertainty" and "chance." Little progress had been made in alleviating the sufferings of mankind.[2] "Why," asked Mary Gove Nichols, "are we sick? Why cannot the doctors cure us?" Men, women, and society had sought a cure so long in vain that they began to distrust their doctors. "We are tired of professions and promises." Mrs. Nichols' solution recalls that of her contemporary, Angenette Hunt: "We ask other help. Let woman be educated. Let her have healthy development . . . if we cannot save the present race, let us raise up a new . . . "[3]

Heroic methods were indeed painful and dangerous, and the American public, sick to death of bloodletting and calomel, rebelled. Occasionally, physicians themselves responded to the crisis with therapeutic nihilism. More often, sectarian practitioners, some with milder and more pleasant forms of treatment, competed successfully for public patronage.

The health reform movement provided a different alternative to a dissatisfied public, and it grew and flourished in the atmosphere created by vociferous debate between sectarians and regulars over more humane methods of treatment. In the early half of the nineteenth century, one begins to discern a gradual shift in the attitudes of men toward sickness and death. The change is not sudden, but it is nevertheless unmistakable. No longer was sickness to be tolerated with the stoicism of the colonials, who tended to leave such decisions in the hands of an often angry and inscrutable God. Slowly, the belief that man could be in greater control of his own destiny, that life and health could be improved through individual effort, replaced the silent resignation of previous generations. The health reform movement encapsulated this transition; the shift is apparent in its vocabulary, its imagery, even in its theory of the origin of disease.

Over and over again health reformers argued that disease was *preventable;* that it was up to the individual to keep himself well. "Many people seem to think that all diseases are immediate visitations from the Almighty, arising from no cause but his *immediate* dispensation," Mary Gove Nichols observed in a book directed specifically to women. "Many seem to have no idea that there are established laws with respect to life and health, and that the transgression of these laws is followed by disease."[4] Her mentor, Sylvester Graham, agreed. Before people attributed disease to a Supreme Being who supposedly loved them, he admonished his readers, they must prove that the cause lies not with their own bad habits.[5] The causes of premature disease and death, declared Marie Louise Shew, wife of the prominent editor of the *Water-Cure Journal,* a popular health reform publication, were mostly within the control of mankind. It is "unwise, irrational, and unphilosophical" to regard illness as the *infliction* of a Divine Providence." It cannot be doubted, she continued, that in accordance with the true designs of

Providence, man was "as a rule" designed to live in good health to a ripe old age.[6] Recent sociologists have pointed out the important connection between the gradual abandonment of passivity and fatalism in the face of life's difficulties, including the willingness to manipulate oneself and one's environment, and the development of the modern personality.[7]

Though health reform advocates came from all the several medical sects and the regulars, their shared theme was the prevention of disease through the teaching of the laws of physiology and hygiene. They accused the regulars of making "no effort to remove the causes of disease," while "vainly" endeavoring "to cure conditions, while causes remain. We even have reason to believe," argued Dr. Ellen M. Snow, "that they have greatly multiplied disease by the use of poisonous drugs." In a chilling denunciation of the dependence of the people on physicians, she declared:

> They do not aim to enlighten mankind in regard to their physical well being, but rather seek to envelop their processes of cure in deep and impenetrable mystery. This mystery possesses a magic charm for the uninitiated and ignorant. You have only to look about you to become aware of the credulity and superstition with which the Medical Profession is regarded. . . .

The health reformer's solemn duty was to "guard the public health"; to "sow far and wide the seeds of truth that will eventually germinate and be the means of redeeming the world from the ignorance that so effectually blinds the mass of its inhabitants."[8]

Such accusations did scant justice to the more forward-looking members of the regular medical profession. Several prominent physicians had long recognized the value of increasing public knowledge of anatomy, physiology, and hygiene. Yet the rhetoric of the health reformers proved more congenial to the public temperament than the somber empiricism of the regulars. Borrowing from the vocabulary of Christian perfectionism to make their point, popular lecturers like Sylvester Graham, William Andrus Alcott, and Mary Gove Nichols succeeded in making health reform a moral imperative.

The concept of self-help was implicit in the health reformers'

theory of sickness. Disease was the remedial effort of Nature to over-
come or cast out of the body some impurity or poison which interfered
with the functions of life.[9] Since the natural condition of man was good
health, to keep well he needed only to avoid unwise practices, such as
eating the wrong foods and losing control of his "passions." Knowledge
of his own physical nature would make man free. "People," announced
Mrs. Shew, "must learn to think for themselves."[10] Ignorance could no
longer be offered as an excuse for illness, agreed Mary Gove Nichols.[11]

Health reformers deplored the complicated language of most
medical journals. "Reader," warned the editor of the *Water-Cure Journal,*
"if you cannot understand what an author is writing about, you may
reasonably presume he does not know himself."[12] "I would have the
highest science, clothed in words, that the people can understand," wrote
Aurelia Raymond, in her graduate thesis at the Female Medical College
of Pennsylvania. "I have studied medicine because I am one of the
people . . . to enter my protest against that exclusiveness, which sets
itself up as something superior to the people. . . ."[13]

Public lectures on physiology and hygiene became an important
tool in the campaign to combat ignorance. In 1837, the American
Physiological Society was founded, an organization of Bostonians
dedicated to the promotion of health and longevity by dispelling
ignorance of physiological laws. William Alcott was the society's first
president, and other prominent health reformers, including Sylvester
Graham and David Cambell, were also involved. During its first year
the society sponsored a number of lectures given by prominent physicians and reformers, including Graham and J.V.C. Smith, the editor of
the highly respected *Boston Medical and Surgical Journal.*[14]

Health reformers emphasized in particular the central role of the
wife and mother in supervising and directing the physiological
regimen—itself a prerequisite to the higher spiritual life. This investment of woman with a special responsibility in the spiritual regeneration of her family, and by extension, of civilization as well, was a
recurring theme in their literature.

Almost one-fourth of the members of the American Physiological
Society were female, and the organization acknowledged the important

role of women in the promotion of good health at its Second Annual Meeting, when the following resolution was passed:

> *Resolved*, That woman in her character as wife and mother is only second to the Deity in the influence that she exerts on the physical, the intellectual and the moral interests of the human race, and that her education should be adapted to qualify her in the highest degree to cherish those interests in the wisest and best manner.[15]

As a result, countless women took to the field as lecturers. In 1838 the newly formed Boston Ladies Physiological Society sponsored a successful and well-publicized series of lectures delivered by Mary Gove Nichols. Before long, similar societies appeared in Providence, Wilmington, Nantucket, Lynn, Bangor, New York, Oberlin, and numerous other towns and cities in the Northeast and West. Nichols, Paulina Wright Davis, Harriot Hunt, Lydia Folger Fowler, and Rachel Brooks Gleason were only a few of the better known of the dozens of women who traveled throughout New England and the West in these decades, teaching other women the "laws of life." Health reform struck a responsive chord in these enthusiastic female audiences. The lecture halls were filled with women eager for the knowledge they hoped would ease their bewilderment with their increased responsibilities within the family—at a time when the home was plagued by pressures imposed from without, by a mobile, fragmented, and fast-changing society.[16] The message of the health reformers seemed an answer, perhaps even a solution, to social instability.

The first half of the nineteenth century witnessed alterations in the economic and social order for which Americans were only minimally prepared. A transportation revolution, and the growth of a national, industrializing economy created a restless society characterized by immense diversity, constant change, and the emergence of new psychological and social roles. Increased social mobility also marked these decades, with individuals moving both upward and downward in social status.

Amidst such change, family patterns were altered. The decline of home industry wrought profound shifts in women's lives. In the colonial period the wife's household duties were a vital contribution to the family's economic survival, but the growth of industry freed her from many important and time-consuming activities, resulting in an increasingly rigid separation between man's and woman's work. Deprived of her economic importance, woman would gradually be required to fulfill a more emotional and ornamental role within the family and society. Many women, however, would seek something more.

Writer and educators incessantly scrutinized the family, examining and re-examining its social role as well as its internal dynamic. During these decades the ideal of the modern family—small in size, emotionally intense, and woman-supervised—first emerged. Americans began to worship the Home, as authors cultivated domesticity at every turn. In a society characterized by instability, the family was idolized as the single potential source for order; it became an enclave, a utopian retreat, a means of escape from excessive freedom and diversity.[17]

All evidence points to a profound concern in these decades for the place, duties, and condition of women. The loss of woman's traditional economic function deprived her role of concrete content, resulting in an obvious decline in morale and autonomy. Yet parallel changes in the first half of the nineteenth century gave women the opportunity to seek alternative outlets for their energies. Religious revivalism notably affected women and increasingly involved them in Moral Reform. Most important, however, the spread of education to women raised their intellectual level and guaranteed the existence of a talented minority with rising status expectations who would feel frustration, distaste, anger, even desperation at the severe limitations imposed on them by the growing popularity of the cult of the "lady." The fashionable, indolent life of the leisured woman was intolerable to those of the emerging middle classes trained in an older Protestant tradition of usefulness, strength, duty, and good works. Gradually there emerged two competing images of the ideal nineteenth century woman, both of which drew strength from the culture which produced them. On the one hand, woman was described as weak, sickly, dependent, and ornamental. On the other she was exalted as highly spiritual and morally superior—confined, for the most part, to the home, yet invested with genuine power and responsibility within her sphere. Both health reformers and women's rights advocates would reject the first and seize upon the second ideal—that of woman's moral power—using it effectively in this century to explore significant and divergent outlets for female energies.[18]

Social fragmentation was costly: it took its toll indiscriminately on society and individual alike. Though earlier generations had faced the problems of an industrializing society in smaller numbers, by the 1830s change had reached crisis proportions. Rarely now could individuals escape its consequences; indeed, an entire society was affected. For some the boundless freedom offered the chance to improve the quality of life for oneself and one's offspring—the options were endless and inviting. For others, however, change was not easy: this was the darker side to limitless opportunity.

For here was a generation prone to illness: sickness, alienation, and fear of physical and psychological collapse proved the response of many to an unfamiliar and too often unsettling historical experience. The hurly burly of urban life seemed especially threatening to some, and countless testimonials in health reform journals warned against the unhealthful environment of city life.[19]

Of particular concern was the state of female health. "If a plan for *destroying female health,* in all the ways in which it could be most effectively done, were drawn up," announced Catherine Beecher, "it would be exactly the course which is now pursued by a large portion of this nation, especially in the more wealthy classes."[20] Augustus K. Gardner, a prominent New York gynecologist, agreed that the present physical condition of women was deplorable.[21] Dr. James C. Jackson of the Dansville water cure unhappily confirmed Gardner's opinion. "American girls," he admitted, "are all sickly."[22] "You are sick," wrote Mrs. S.M. Estee to the feminine readers of the *Water-Cure Journal,* "and have been for months, years, and some of you your whole lives."[23]

We cannot know for sure, of course, whether or not this generation of women was sicker than their grandmothers. What is certain, however, is that they *thought* they were. Indeed, they may very well have been. Fashionable dress took its toll on female health as more and more women moved into the middle class; in particular, the corset and tight lacing did much damage to female anatomy. Increased urbanization and the decline of home industry meant that more and more women would be denied the fresh air and vigorous exercise enjoyed of necessity by the rural housewife. And the psychological strains of dislocation may have prompted some women to opt for ill-health rather than stand and face changes they could still barely comprehend.[24]

Health reform offered to countless women a means of coping with an imprecise, undependable, and often hostile environment. In a society in which women were expected to play an increasingly complex role in the nurture of children and the organization of family life, health reform brought to the bewildered housewife not just sympathy and compassion, but a structured regimen, a way of life. In an era characterized by weakening ties between relatives and neighbors, health reform lectures, journals, and domestic tracts provided once again the friendly advice and companionship of the now remote kinswoman. Women were promised a means to end their isolation and make contact with others of their sex. At lectures, study groups, and even through letters to the various journals, they shared their common experiences with other women. A deep sense of sisterhood was evidenced by the frequent use of the term. No longer must woman bear her burden alone.

Health reform was one means by which many women articulated their feminism, and these reformers understood the importance of good health as a prerequisite for woman's place in the world. "Woman was neither made a toy nor a slave, but a help-meet to man," wrote "A Bloomer to Her Sisters," "and as such devolves upon her very many important duties and obligations, which cannot be met so long as she is the puny, sickly, aching, weakly, dying creature that we find her to be; and woman must, to a very considerable extent, redeem herself—she must throw off the shackles that have hitherto bound both body and mind, and rise into the newness of life."[25]

Health reformers were acutely conscious of the fact that woman was in the process of creating for herself a new role. "Woman . . . is a new element in society," wrote James C. Jackson to Harriet A. Judd, M.D., "just emerging from her hybernation . . . and so much better fitted to take to herself *new* ideas, and develop them. . . ."[26] Good health was essential to woman's new self-expression, equality, and improved status. "Let mothers be educated in all that concerns life and health . . ." insisted Mrs. Eliza de La Vergue, M.D. "*Let them learn that knowledge gives the highest order of power.*"[27] Harriet Austin thought speculation on woman's sphere a waste of time. "It is her sphere," she insisted, "to do what she desires to do." When, she continued, "conscious of the divinity within her," and "of the mightiness of her power" she determines to elevate, not only her sex, but humanity, this too will be her sphere. "But," warned Miss Austin, "this work can never be accomplished while woman remains sick." Woman's sphere could not be expanded until she "learns and claims her first great right—the right to health."[28]

Far from an eccentric fad, dress reform became a principal element in the health reformers' program for women. Health reformers were not the only ones who understood the connection between fashionable dress and female ill-health; occasionally regular physicians were themselves outspoken on the matter. But the health reformers succeeded in making dress reform a moral imperative, and they connected dress reform to feminist aspirations. They made it clear that good health could never come as long as women clung to the immoral dictates of French fashion, and they called upon women to liberate their souls by freeing their bodies from the harmful effects of tight lacing and long, heavy, unhygienic skirts. "How . . . glorious," mused Rachel Brooks Gleason, M.D., "would it be to see every woman free from *every* fetter that fashion has imposed! Such a day of 'universal emancipation' of the sex would be worthy of a celebration through all coming time."[29] "We can expect but small achievement from women," warned Mary Gove Nichols, "so long as it is the labor of their lives to carry about their clothes."[30] "How in the name of common sense," agreed Edith Denner, "is a woman with long, full skirts, ever to become a practical Ornithologist, Geologist, or Botanist . . . without a great deal of inconvenience, attended by a vast amount of unnecessary labor and fatigue?"[31]

Reform journals pressed the issue incessantly. Lengthy technical descriptions of the damage wreaked on female anatomy by the corset appeared, complete with diagrams. Pictures of the "Allopathic Lady, or 'Pure Cod Liver Oil Female,' Who Patronizes a Fashionable Doctor, And Considers It Decidedly Vulgar to Enjoy Good Health," were published side by side with those of women in reformed dress, under which the caption read "A Water-Cure Bloomer, Who Believes In The

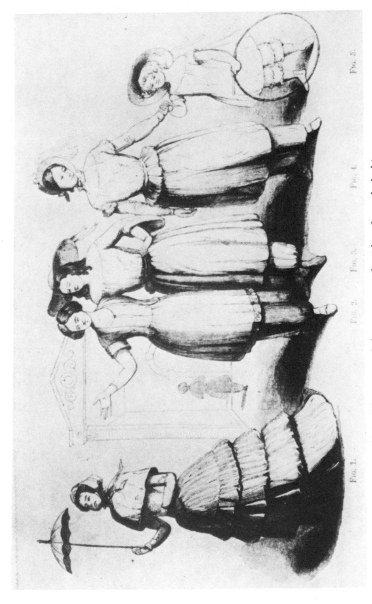

Fashionable corseted dress compared with reformed clothing. Illustration in the *Water-Cure Journal* 12, No. 2, August 1851, p. 36.

Equal Rights of Men And Women To Help Themselves And Each Other, And Who Thinks It Respectable, If Not Genteel, To Be Well."[32] Not content merely to admonish their readers, some journals printed sewing instructions to make the reformed dress; the *Laws of Life* sold patterns of the "American Costume" to its female readers.[33]

Health reformers were perfectionists, and they saw in the improvement of the individual a means of social regeneration. Nothing less than the future of civilization was at stake, and health reformers gave to woman a new importance and purpose by emphasizing her central and positive role in the task of human betterment. As the concern to maintain social order in a mobile, urbanizing, and industrializing society became acute, thinkers and educators turned their hopes to the family, assigning to it the task of creating responsible adults— individuals who could impose their own private structure on an imprecise, undependable society. The investment of home and domesticity with supreme significance was an essential ingredient in the transformation of woman's role, and health reform both reflected and contributed to this larger cultural theme.

As early as 1839, William A. Alcott, in his book *The Young Mother,* took for granted the mother's primary responsibility in child-rearing and the father's extended absence from the home.

> Let it be left to the fathers to study the improvements of hounds and horses and cattle, and at the same time think themselves above the concerns of the nursery. . . . But our passion for gain, in the present age is so much more absorbing and soul destroying. . . . Oh no. All, or nearly all, must devolve on the mother. The father has no time to attend to his children.[34]

Much of the information in health reform literature, both practical and prescriptive, was consequently directed at woman in her capacity as wife and mother. She was invested with awesome responsibilities. "There are no duties on earth so nearly angelic as those which devolve upon woman . . . ," declared Alcott. "If all wives loved and delighted in their homes as Solomon would have them, few husbands would go down to a premature grave through the avenues of intemperance and lust, and their kindred vices."[35]

The Lily, a feminist and temperance journal, emphasized woman's moral power. "Woman's influence is truly kingly [*sic*] in general society. It is powerful in a daughter and a sister; but it is the mother who weaves the garlands that flourish in eternity."[36] The gravity of woman's influence went even beyond her own family, for health reformers shared a widespread contemporary belief in the inheritance of acquired characteristics.[37] "For the sake of the race," explained Mary Gove Nichols, "I ask that all be done for woman that can be done, for it is an awful truth that fools are the mothers of fools." Elsewhere she observed that "the civilized world is full of sick women. This is the mighty evil that now overshadows the world. It must be removed, or mankind has no future."[38] James C. Jackson was even more blunt: "God punishes as well as rewards mankind *through woman*. . . . She is appointed to dispense divine retributions as well as divine blessings. . . . through her does God visit the iniquities of the father on the children to the third and fourth generations."[39]

Though such attitudes gave to women genuine responsibility and power, they also exacted a large measure of anxiety and even guilt. "Women are answerable, in a very large degree," admonished Paulina Wright Davis, "for the imbecilities of disease, mental and bodily, and for the premature deaths prevailing throughout society—for the weakness, wretchedness, and shortness of life—and no remedy will be radical till reformation of life and practice obtains among our sex. . . ."[40]

Such a psychological burden might well have been unbearable had not health reformers offered women fellowship, moral support, and practical information. "I wish," wrote Mary Gove Nichols of her motives in becoming a health reformer, "to teach mothers how to cure their own diseases, and those of their children; and to increase health, purity, and happiness in the family and the home."[41]

For some women, at least, Mrs. Nichols and her fellow reformers achieved these goals. Numerous articles on cookery, bathing, teething, care of infants, childhood sexuality, cleanliness, and domestic economy carefully taught women how to manage their households properly. Itinerant physiological lecturers assaulted women's widespread ignorance of their bodies. Mrs. Nichols, for example, relied heavily on a discussion of anatomy and physiology in her lectures. She instructed her listeners in the formation of bone structure, the role of respiration and circulation, the anatomy and physiology of the stomach. The process of digestion was described in detail. The remainder of her course involved information on dietetics and the importance of physical education. The evils of "tight lacing," and dire warnings against the harmful effects of the "solitary vice" also proved popular topics for discussion.

Advice on the supervision of pregnancy and childbirth was surprisingly modern. Whereas regular physicians still treated pregnancy and childbirth as a disease—often drugging both mother and infant—health reformers insisted that both be welcomed as natural events, urging exercise without fatigue, fresh air, proper diet, and cleanliness. Daily bathing for infants was suggested and they were to be dressed in loose-fitting garments to give plenty of opportunity for movement. To hinder chafing, sweet oil rubbed in the creases of the flesh was advised. No drugs were allowed for mother or child.[42] It is hardly surprising that such attention to hygiene and diet actually improved the health of many, a fact attested to by numerous testimonials from satisfied individuals to be found in the back pages of health reform journals.[43]

Acknowledging the positive influence of woman in society and the family led some health reformers to a re-examination of the relationship between the sexes. During these years many of them openly rejected the older authoritarian concept of marriage in favor of a relationship based on mutual love, common interest, and affection. Men were urged to pattern themselves after their wives, whereas women were told to imitate the strength and conviction of their husbands. Groping toward a redefinition of masculinity and femininity, James C. Jackson observed,

> while it never looks well to see a *masculine* woman, or an *effeminate* man, it *does* look well to see a *manly* woman, and a *feminine* man, the one wearing over her delicacy decision and consciousness of purpose, the other over his massive strength, those soft and kindly touchings which polish but weaken not, yet rather serve to give his essential characteristics thorougher relief.[44]

Sexual purity before marriage was now to be required of both sexes, and the double standard was deplored. Restraint in sexual matters promoted physical and spiritual health, and woman's presumed lack of sexual feeling was held up as the ideal. Fathers were urged to forsake the pursuit of money and reinvolve themselves in the wholesome atmosphere of family life; the spiritual rewards of parenthood were emphasized.[45] Married couples should learn to share each other's concerns. Indeed, the pursuit of a "companionate marriage" led many young men and women to advertise for like-minded mates in the *Water-Cure Journal,* which for a number of years devoted an entire section to matrimonial advertising. One such ad, placed by "Henry Homes" paints a congenial and inviting scene of the mutuality inherent in the reformers' ideal of domestic life:

> I seek a congenial spirit, if she is of the EARNEST, BRAVE, and TRUE, with well developed brain and body, a warm heart, and willing hand; in other words, INTELLIGENT, SYMPATHIZING, and PRACTICAL. Am 22, medium height, size of brain 23 inches; temperament, nervous-sanguine; a RADICAL thinker and truth seeker, with untrammeled mind; anti-rum, slavery, drug, tea, and coffee, and am a vegetarian; am identified with the cause of human progress; a great lover of home, and warmly attached to friends, and those who cherish my sentiments. Shall be happy to communicate with any one interested. Address Greenville, Darke County, Ohio.

Women advertised as well, and the picture would not be complete without a typical feminine request for a husband: "I am thirty years old," wrote Victoria,

> five feet two inches high, healthy, and considered good looking, black hair and eyes, weigh 150 lbs; am just the one that knows when the household duties are done right or not; can spin, weave, teach school, and if necessary work in the meadow, too; am economical in all matters, I think; am anti-slavery, temperance, and a strong believer in phrenology, hydropathy, and advocate the rights of women, and have adopted the Bloomer dress . . . will exchange miniatures if requested. . . .[46]

Victoria would not have mixed well with a group of fashionable nineteenth century ladies. It was just such an ineffective and ornamental role for women that health reformers repeatedly deplored.

Once the conception of woman as the moral arbiter of society gained an audience, the ideal itself became a potent source for social change. Involvement in health reform was one means by which countless women could widen their sphere by moving out into society. The most logical extension of the health reformers assessment of woman's natural abilities was to teach women medicine. Indeed, the entrance of women into the medical profession grew out of the health reform movement. "In sickness there is no hand like a woman's hand," the *Water-Cure Journal* reminded its readers.[47] "The property of her nature," argued a contributor to *Godey's Lady's Book,* "which renders her the best of nurses, with proper instruction, equally qualifies her to be the best of physicians. Above all is this the case with her own sex and her children."[48] Enthusiastically, health reformers applauded the acceptance of women as medical students, chiding the regulars for their conservatism. "What," asked the editor of the *Water-Cure Journal,* "will our Allopathic doctors say to this? We pause for a reply. In the meantime, our women are buckling on the armor for a struggle which must ultimately prove successful."[49] In time these pioneer women physicians, who were attracted to medicine out of an ardent desire to fulfill their destinies as superior moral beings with natural abilities to cure, would be transformed into full-fledged professionals by their contact with an increasingly scientific and empirical discipline. They, as well as their system of values, would be permanently altered in the process.

The health reform movement flourished in the mid-nineteenth century largely because of the simultaneous occurrence of two historical events: the failure of heroic medicine to cure, and the emergence of a modern personality type for whom such a situation was intolerable. Health reform was both cause *and* effect in the process, in the sense that it embodied the revolt against traditional authority in medical matters and the rejection of stoicism in the face of disease, while offering to individuals a temporarily viable alternative to the painful and dangerous therapeutics of the old school.

To women health reform gave even more. Developing a coherent program designed to cope with both the physical and psychological burdens imposed by a society in transition, it held out to confused wives and mothers the prospect of improving the quality of life, not by changing the environment, but by gaining control of oneself. It promised women that they would raise their children healthy in mind and clean in body. It offered to them the possibility of keeping their husbands moral by cooking the right foods. Preaching sexual continence and physiological knowledge, health reformers helped legitimate the rights of women in sexual matters at a time when sexual contact was not necessarily a positive experience for many women. Health manuals aided women in dealing with sexuality in themselves, their husbands, and their children. Emphasizing woman's essential role as teacher and spiritual arbiter within the family, health reform literature contributed to the enhancement of woman's status at a time when cultural and economic changes had obscured her role and narrowed her usefulness. And though this investment of the womanly sphere with cosmic moral significance was a broader cultural trend, shared by the society as a whole, health reformers, unlike many nineteenth century thinkers, subscribed to the widest possible definition of woman's sphere. They understood full well that to purify society, women would indeed have to enter it. Thus, for some brave, ambitious, and talented women, health reform provided an outlet and an escape from an intolerably narrow and confining role.

Moving out into the world, women transformed society's conception of the duties and abilities of the female sex, while they themselves were also changed. Health reform marked a hitherto unexplored historical step on the tortuous road to full equality for women. How little did she divine the far-reaching implications of her words, when Mrs. S.M. Estee of the Petersburg Water Cure attempted to inspire her "sick sisters" with the following:

> Cheer up, ye sick and drooping! there is a panacea for your ills; it is not to be found in poisonous drugs, but in heaven's pure air, the soft, refreshing water that issues bubbling from the hill-sides, appropriate exercise, and proper diet; then cheer up, ye disconsolate ones! and be assured there is a balm in Gilead, and there are true physicians.[50]

References

*The author is grateful to Bill Chafe, Ellen Chesler, Judy Leavitt, and Ron Walters, whose suggestions helped clarify her thinking on several points.

[1] Ann Preston, "General Diagnosis," 1851; Angenette A. Hunt, "The True Physician," 1851. Theses in Medical College of Pennsylvania Archives (MCP).

[2] Marie Louise Shew, *Water Cure for Ladies: A Popular Work on the Health Diet and Regimen of Females and Children,* revised by Joel Shew, M.D. (New York: Wiley & Putnam, 1844), pp. 20, 23.

[3] Angenette Hunt, "Woman the Physician," *Water-Cure Journal* 11(1851): 74-75. Hereafter cited as *WCJ*.

[4] Mary S. Gove [Nichols], *Lectures to Women on Anatomy and Physiology* (New York: Harper and Brothers, 1846), p. 20.

[5] William Applegate, *A Defense of the Graham System of Living* (New York: W. Applegate, 1835), p. 23.

[6] M.L. Shew, *Water Cure for Ladies,* pp. 14, 15. See also Mary Gove Nichols, *A Woman's Work in Water Cure and Sanitary Education* (London: Nichols, 1874), p. 80.

[7] See especially Richard D. Brown, "Modernization and the Modern Personality in America, 1600-1865," *Journal of Interdisciplinary History* 2(1972): 201-227; Alex Inkeles, "Making Men Modern: On the Causes and Consequences of Individual Change in Six Developing Countries," *American Journal of Sociology* 75(1969): 210.

[8] "Duties of Physicians," *WCJ* 21(1856): 55-56.

[9] See Thomas L. Nichols, *Eating to Live: The Diet Cure* (New York: M.L. Holbrook & Co., 1881); also *WCJ* 25(1858): 53, an article by Dr. N. Bedortha of the Saratoga Springs water cure in which this general view was somewhat modified.

[10] Shew, *Water Cure for Ladies,* Preface, p. iii.

[11] Nichols, *A Woman's Work in Water Cure,* p. 80.

[12] "Old School Medical Journals," *WCJ* 9(1850): 181.

[13] Aurelia Raymond, "Thesis on the Human Brain," 1864, thesis in MCP Archives.

[14] See Hebbel E. Hoff, M.D., and John F. Fulton, M.D., "The Centenary of the First American Physiological Society," *Bulletin of the History of Medicine* 5(October 1939): 687-733.

[15] *Ibid.,* p. 701.

[16] *Library of Health* 2(1838): 70, 367; 6(1842): 156; 5(1841): 40; Thomas L. Nichols, *Health Manual: Being Also A Memorial of the Life and Work of Mrs. Mary S. Gove Nichols* (London: Allen, 1887), p. 22; *WCJ* 1(1846), 11(1851): 29, 38, 93; 9(1850): 90; 14(1852): 56; 17(1854): 46; 22(1856): 131; 28(1859): 57-58; 5(1848): 83; *Graham Journal* II(1838): 37, 181, 288, 385; III(1839): 20, 37, 82; *The Lily* III(1851): 27. *The Una* I(1854): 206; II(1854): 263; *Boston Medical and Surgical Journal* 40(1849): 107, 48(1853): 443-444.

[17] For secondary sources on social and economic change in this period see Robert Fogel and Stanley Engerman, eds., *The Reinterpretation of Economic History,* (New York: Harper & Row, 1971); Stephan Thernstrom, *Poverty and Progress,* (Cambridge: Harvard University Press, 1964). Three helpful works on the family are: Kirk Jeffrey, "The Family as a Utopian Retreat from the City," *Soundings* (Spring 1972): 21-41; Kirk Jeffrey, "Family History: The Middle-Class American Family in the Urban Context, 1830-1870," Ph.D. thesis, Stanford University, 1971; Mary P. Ryan, "American Society and the Cult of Domesticity," Ph.D. thesis, University of California at Santa Barbara, 1971.

[18] See Keith Melder, "The Beginning of the Women's Rights Movement in the United States, 1800-1840," Ph.D. thesis, Yale University, 1964; and Gerda Lerner, "The Lady and the Mill Girl: Changes in the Status of Women in the Age of Jackson," *American Studies Journal* 10(Spring 1969): 5-15.

[19] See Stephen Nissenbaum, "Careful Love; Sylvester Graham and the Emergence of Victorian Sexual Theory in America, 1830-1840," Ph.D. thesis, University of Wisconsin, 1968; Stephen Nissenbaum, "Sex, Reform and Social Change, 1830-1840," unpublished paper delivered at the 1972 meeting of the Organization of American Historians.

[20] Catharine Beecher, *Letters to the People on Health and Happiness* (New York, 1856), p. 7.

[21] Reprinted from the *Knickerbocker Journal, WCJ* 29(1860): 21-22, 50-51.

[22] James C. Jackson, "Shall Our Girls Live or Die?" *Laws of Life* 10(1867): 2.

[23] Mrs. S.M. Estee, "To Sick Women," *WCJ* 26(1858): 96. Many well-known feminists, including Lucy Stone, Catherine Beecher, Elizabeth Smith Miller, Angelina Grimke, and Susan B. Anthony, were plagued by chronic illness. Most of them were interested in health reform.

[24] See Carroll Smith-Rosenberg, "The Hysterical Woman: Sex Roles and Role Conflict in Nineteenth-Century America," *Social Research* 39(Winter 1972): 652-678.

[25] Sarah E. Selby, "A Bloomer to her Sisters," *WCJ* 15(1853): 131.

[26] *WCJ* 15(1854): 74, 94.

[27] Italics mine. Mrs. Eliza de la Vergue, M.D., *WCJ* 20(1855): 74.

[28] Harriet Austin, "Woman's Present and Future," *WCJ* 16(1853): 57.

[29] Mrs. R.B. Gleason, M.D., "Woman's Dress," *WCJ* 11(1851): 30.

[30] Mary Gove Nichols, "The New Costume," *WCJ* 12(1851): 30.

[31] Edith Denner, "Science and Long Skirts," *WCJ* 20(1855): 7.

[32] See *WCJ* 16(1853): 120; and 11(1851): 96, and passim.

[33] Dress reform was also a popular topic in women's rights journals like *The Una, The Lily,* and later *The Revolution.* Many of the articles in these journals pertaining to dress were written by health reformers. See especially *WCJ* 12(1851): 33, 58; *WCJ* 34(1862): 1-2; *WCJ* 15(1853): 7, 10, 32, 34, 35, 131; *WCJ* 13(1852): 111; *The Laws of Life* 10(1867): 93-94, 129-130, 145-146; *The Revolution* 3(1869): 149-150; *Graham Journal* 3(1839): 301-302.

[34] William A. Alcott, *The Young Mother* (Boston: G. W. Light, 1839), pp. 265-266.

[35] William A. Alcott, *The Young Wife,* (Boston: G. W. Light, 1837), pp. 87-89.

[36] *The Lily* I(1849): 52.

[37] For an excellent summary of hereditarian views in this period, see Charles Rosenberg, "The Bitter Fruit: Heredity, Disease, and Social Thought in Nineteenth-Century America," *Perspectives in American History* 7(1974): 189-238.

[38] Nichols, *Lectures to Women,* p. 212. Mary Gove Nichols, "Woman the Physician," *WCJ* 12(1851): 75.

[39] James C. Jackson, "The Women of the United States," *WCJ* 26(1858): 3. Also, James C. Jackson, "Women's Rights," *WCJ* 31(1861): 61.

[40] Paulina Wright Davis, *WCJ* 1(1846): 29.

[41] Nichols, *A Woman's Work in Water Cure*, p. 14.

[42] See especially, Thomas L. Nichols, *"The Curse Removed": A Statement of Facts Respecting the Efficacy of Water-Cure in the Treatment of Uterine Diseases and the Removal of the Pains and Perils of Pregnancy and Childbirth* (New York: The Water-Cure Journal, 1850); M.G. Nichols, "Maternity; and the Water Cure of Infants," *WCJ* 11(1851): 57-59; *Graham Journal,* "Keep Your Children Clean," I(1837): 176; "Masturbation and Its Effect on Health," II(1838): 23. Mary Gove Nichols, *Lectures to Women,* passim. See also advertisement in the *Graham Journal* II(1838): 288. For articles on fresh air and bathing: *WCJ* 3(1847): 161-168, 177; *WCJ* 4(1847): 193; pregnancy, exercise, and childbirth: *WCJ* 3(1847): 145, 151, 183-184; "Our New Cookbook," "How to Can a Fruit," *Laws of Life* 10(1867): 12; "Cleanliness and Healthfulness," *Laws of Life* 10(1867): 16; "Teething and its Management," "Children's Dress," *WCJ* 12(1851): 101, 104.

[43] See an interesting autobiographical sketch by Mrs. Mary A. Torbit, "Reasons for Becoming a Lecturer," *WCJ* 14(1852): 91.

[44] James C. Jackson, *WCJ* 22(1856): 40.

[45] Nissenbaum, "Sylvester Graham," *Godey's Lady's Book* 55(1857): 47. Elizabeth Blackwell would incessantly press this point. See especially, "Criticism of Gronlund's Cooperative Commonwealth, Chapter X—Women," n.d., pp. 9-11, Blackwell MSS, Library of Congress. Also, "A Thought on Social Relations," *Laws of Life* 10(1867): 10.

[46] See *WCJ* 21(1856): 23; *WCJ* 20(1855): 95; *WCJ* 17(1854): 11; *WCJ* 26(1856): 96.

[47] "Woman's Tenderness and Love," *WCJ* 5(1848): 95.

[48] William M. Cornell, M.D., "Woman the True Physician," *WCJ* 46(1853): 82.

[49] *WCJ* 12(1851): 73-75; M.G. Nichols, "Woman, the Physician," *WCJ* 12(1851): 73-75; "Female Physicians," *The Lily* I(1849): 94; II(1850): 39, 70, 77; "Female Physicians," *WCJ* 31(1861): 84; Augusta R. Montgomery, "The Medical Education of Women," 1853, thesis, MCP Archives; *Godey's Lady's Book* 44(1852): 185-189; 61(1860): 270-271; 54(1857): 371; 49(1854): 80, 368, 456; *The Revolution* I(1868): 170, 201, 339; III(1870): 252; *WCJ* 13(1852): 34-35, 86-87; 29(1860): 45, 2-3; 31(1861): 42; 28(1859): 84.

[50] Estee, "To Sick Women," *WCJ* 26(1858): 96.

Patent Medicines
and the Self-Help Syndrome

James Harvey Young

"Somebody buys all the quack medicines," Oliver Wendell Holmes once wrote, "that build palaces for the mushroom, say rather, the toadstool millionaires."[1] To comprehend the kind of medical self-help that involves the use of patent medicines, therefore, we need to try to understand both parties to the transaction, the seller of the nostrums and that "somebody" who buys them.

Both seller and buyer possess complex and subtle motives; hence the task of comprehension is not easy. In his public face, advertising, the seller most often disguises or distorts his most obvious aim. And patent medicine promoters have on the whole protected their privacy with great diligence. They have in the main eschewed the art of autobiography. When biographical information has appeared, in book or magazine, it too often sounds like a mere extension of advertising. Few documented histories of proprietary medicine companies exist.[2]

Nor, on the buyer side, do we have an abundance of conscious, candid self-revelation. Proprietary users do not keep diaries of their medicine-taking habits in which they detail their symptoms and analyze their motives for purchasing a given pill or potion. So we must try to recapture the experience from piecing together evidence from the kinds of records that do exist.

Voltaire said that quackery began when the first knave met the first fool. Throughout most of history quackery has principally involved face-to-face encounter, so that the quack's presence—his personality, costume, oratory, showmanship—have overwhelmed the customer-victim. He might be selling a potion, an amulet, or a laying on of his powerful hands. Responding to the overawed reaction of those to whom he ministered, the quack often became as persuaded as did they, however unscrupulous his initial motives, that his drug, device, or manipulation possessed healing power. For, as Grete de Francesco has written, "The charlatan resembled his dupes; his, too, was a weak and disappointed nature that sought compensation in the realm of illusion, on a plane that was no longer that of the sober earth."[3] Thus both parties to the transaction could be enveloped in delusion.

Face-to-face quackery still flourishes, the quack dispensing drugs with polysyllabic chemical names, vitamins lettered far down into the alphabet, treatments with complex and impressive machines, and the laying on of hands, all done with glowing therapeutic promises. To the patient-victim it makes no difference whether his self-asserted savior lies brazenly or speaks what he himself ignorantly believes to be the truth.

Patent medicines—and devices similarly promoted—separate the proprietor from the user by one or more removes and owe their origin to the more complex and sophisticated modes of life ushered in by the commercial and the printing revolutions. Printing created the newspaper, and seventeenth century English journals quickly blossomed forth with nostrum ads. *Mercurius Politicus* during 1660, for example, touted a dentifrice which would make the teeth "white as Ivory," fasten them firmly, prevent toothache, sweeten the breath, and banish cankers.[4] The ad gave a location at which customers could buy this wonder, the shop of a stationer beside St. Paul's Church. Presumably the stationer was middleman, not the dentifrice maker himself. If such a proprietor could place his product in various London shops, as well as in shops throughout the countryside, a feat which better transportation had made easier, and could lure customers into those shops by means of printed advertising, he had expanded his potential market tremendously over that possible through face-to-face appeals. Competition developed so rapidly in this new favorable environment that, to distinguish his product from its many rivals, a promoter endowed it with badges of proprietorship, especially a container of unique design, often pictured in newspaper advertising.[5]

The evolving patent system began, during the early eighteenth century, to cover compound medicines. Proprietors who chose to patent their formulas boasted that this step signified governmental endorsement of therapeutic efficacy. In exchange for the dubious right to make this false claim, those securing patents had to reveal each medicine's composition. Most proprietors preferred to vend secret formulas without a patent. The term "patent medicine" came in common parlance to apply to both categories indistinguishably.

English patent medicines appear on the American market early in the eighteenth century, advertised soon after the origin of the colonial press. By mid-century such advertising had become abundant, continuing to expand until tensions between colony and mother country put restrictions on trade. An odd circumstance differentiates the advertising of the same brands of patent medicines in the British and in the American press. In England the nostrum proprietor sought to transfer into print something of the high-flown harangue used by quacks in face-to-face promotion, often using for the purpose several column inches of type. In colonial America this hardly ever happened. Only a few hyperbolic pamphlets extolling the virtues of patent remedies have come down to us, and only with great rarity in the late colonial years did a nostrum ad appear smacking of the customary British vim and vigor. For the most part, colonial advertisements of the British patent medicines consist of mere names in lists. The latest ship from London had come to port, so Anderson's Scots Pills, Bateman's Pectoral Drops, Hooper's Female Pills and other familiar name-brands were now available. Customers in colonial towns bought patent medicines from many outlets; apothecaries, booksellers, goldsmiths, grocers, hairdressers, tailors, and printers—among other tradesmen—vended them.

Why the terse, drab American advertising? For one thing, remoteness of the proprietors. Busy competing with each other at home, they had not extended their technique of grandiose promotion across the ocean. As a consequence, the American weeklies, modest in size, had not been pushed to expand advertising space so as to rival that in the more frequent and numerous English newspapers. On the American side, perhaps the medicines sold well enough without the British harangues in print. Supply may never have exceeded demand so markedly in the colonies as in the mother country. Certainly Americans lacked initiative in creating nostrums to compete with the traditional British brands, for only rarely, to judge from the press, did some colonist move an eye-water or a salve from the realm of folk medicine into commerce.[6] Americans became accustomed to dosing themselves with the British brands—many physicians prescribed them—and out of a sense of tradition and loyalty continued to use them. Indeed, when political loyalty began to wear thin, medicinal loyalty persisted, for customers so desired the brand-name British nostrums now cut off by economic warfare, that American apothecaries refilled empty bottles by the gross.

Patent medicines shared in the burst of creativity let loose by the cultural nationalism of the Revolutionary generation. Made-in-America nostrums proliferated, a few of them patented when the Constitution authorized this protection to inventors, but most of them shrouded in secrecy. Competition increased and proprietors bought ever more space in the burgeoning newspapers to acclaim their own respective brands. In time, joining nationalism as a stimulating force, came the thrust for an expansion of democracy. Physicians came under suspicion because of their "heroic" bleeding and purging, a battle in which Thomsonians[7] and homeopaths were joined by patent medicine makers who boasted to an increasingly worried public about how painless, nice-tasting, and non-mineral their proprietary products were as compared with the regular doctors' lancet and mercury.[8]

Learned physicians also lost caste, along with members of other educated professions, during the cultural climate associated with Jacksonian democracy. As leaders of opinion lost this traditional role, each common man had to make up his own mind for himself. The right to do so stimulates pride, fires ambition, but also provokes anxiety. Which of the many new voices appealing for favor can be believed? Hard, sharp, unscrupulous bargaining reigns in the realms of both thought and trade. Life becomes intensely competitive. A horde of tricksters appears. Victimization runs rampant. Everybody expects roguery, anticipates being cheated, himself cheats in turn. Nor, within limits, do people mind being hoodwinked. They have made their own decisions, taken their chances in a free environment. Sometimes they are bound to lose. Indeed, clever imposture amuses them. Such a picture of the popular mind emerges from Neil Harris' brilliant book on "the art of P.T. Barnum," entitled *Humbug.*[9]

In this pervasive atmosphere of caveat emptor, American patent medicines soared. Becoming more literate through the expansion of

elementary schooling, citizens read newspaper advertising and deter-
mined on their own which nostrums to buy in order to treat their
ailments. Much advertising explicitly attacked the high-and-mighty
arrogance of regular physicians. Whatever affliction bothered the
common man, patent medicines promised a cure for it. Cholera remedies proliferated during epidemics, and year-in year-out concern for
tuberculosis received constant prodding in advertising columns. That so
many nostrums contained laxative ingredients gives insight into the
poor dietary habits of the mid-nineteenth century. Constipation, indeed, appeared in much patent medicine advertising as a grim harbinger
of worse ills to come. To judge from advertising also, Americans led
dreary, boring, work-filled, depressing lives, and many nostrums, some
containing alcohol, fell into a sort of "mood drug" category.

One such mood drug may be used for more extended illustration,
not because it completely typifies nineteenth century patent medicine
promotion—each case history has its unique particulars—but because it
reveals several significant features of the way proprietary medicines
intertwined with broader facets of life.

When the panic of 1873 struck the nation, Mrs. Lydia Estes
Pinkham had attained the age of 54. For thirty years she had struggled to
maintain her family of three sons and a daughter—another son had died
in infancy—on the hope that one of her husband Isaac's many specula-
tions, mainly in real estate, might handsomely pay off. None had done
so, and the depression ended all such hope and snuffed out Isaac's will to
strive. In family council, Lydia and her sons took things into their own
hands.[10]

Like many enterprising housewives, Lydia for years had nursed
members of her family when they were ill, using remedies remembered
from family tradition and gathered from medical guides which she liked
to read. A particular favorite of hers, John King's *American Dispensatory,*
fell into that class of popular botanical handbooks stemming from the
revived interest in the vegetable kingdom stimulated by Thomsonianism. Lydia Pinkham, a good neighbor, dosed others outside her family
when they were ailing. Strangers sometimes showed up at her door
asking for her concoctions which they had heard about in conversation.
For centuries, folklore remedies, administered gratis by grandmothers

and maiden aunts, had occasionally become articles for sale under the press of financial exigency. Now in the Pinkham household the need indeed was great, and one of Lydia's favorite vegetable brews became a proprietary medicine.

The bottles filled in the Pinkham cellar kitchen in Lynn, Massachusetts, contained not only a mixture of several botanicals but a fillip of reform. For Lydia had grown up amidst freedom's ferment and had shown strong interest in many causes. Her parents had left their Friends meeting over the issue of slavery, and Lydia herself embraced strong abolitionist sentiments, belonging to the Female Anti-Slavery Society and developing an acquaintance with Garrison, Whittier, Frederick Douglass, Abby Kelley, the Grimké sisters, and other abolitionist worthies. Lydia espoused temperance, even though her Vegetable Compound was to contain 18 percent alcohol. She looked with favor on the food reform doctrines of Sylvester Graham, supported inflation through the issuance of greenbacks, welcomed phrenology, and believed with increasing intensity in spiritualism. Lydia helped establish and served as secretary for the Freeman's Institute, a group formed for the uninhibited discussion of all social ideas.

So, of course, living in this climate, Lydia believed in a larger role for women in society. As Samuel Thomson's system had sought to strike a blow for medical democracy, so Lydia E. Pinkham's Vegetable Compound sought to strike a blow for woman's rights. Lydia had developed the belief that male physicians were insensitive to women's ills.[11] When testimonials began arriving in the mail praising her new proprietary, they confirmed her own conviction. "I had doctored with the physicians of this town for three years," read one such letter, "and grew worse instead of better." Lydia hoped for a more tolerant attitude than that which then prevailed toward women seeking to become doctors, and she clipped newspaper stories relating to women and medical education. Her own role with respect to women's health would be different but, as she saw it, no less important. She would bottle and sell the vegetable compound she had adapted from King's *Dispensatory* and had prescribed for women of her acquaintance who had seemed pleased with the results.

"Only a woman understands a woman's ills," Lydia believed, and

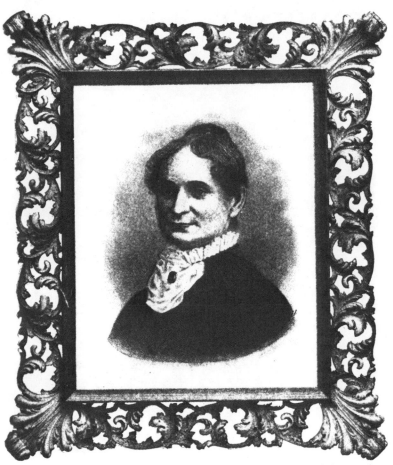

Lydia E. Pinkham.

this maxim became an advertising slogan, as her own dignified grey-haired countenance became her remedy's trademark. Soon her advertising urged women to write her for advice about their most intimate health problems, promising that no male eye would see the letters. For a while she penned the answers herself, but soon the pressure of work caused her to introduce other female relatives to this task, the advice now dictated to women stenographers skilled at using that new invention, the typewriter. Lydia's letters urged the use of her Compound, but also gave counsel on diet, dress, and bathing. "Keep clean inside and out" was a favorite injunction. Most letters evidently employed the imperative mode.

In the nineteenth century any lay person could do just what Lydia Pinkham did, devise a formula inspired or informed by whatever sources of information came to hand, and market the medicine with whatever therapeutic claims seemed likely to persuade. The marketplace groaned with packages of inert ingredients ballyhooed as cures for cancer and with opium-laden syrups vended to soothe fretful babies. Lydia Pinkham exercised more restraint than most of her fellow competitors in proprietary marketing. She had the support of eclectic medicine for most of the ingredients in her Vegetable Compound and for many of her claims. King's *American Dispensatory* praised the true unicorn root—her mixture also contained the false unicorn root—for "the tonic influence it exerts upon the female generative organs, giving a normal energy to the uterus, and thus proving helpful in cases where there is an habitual tendency to miscarriage."[12] King also asserted that pleurisy root had helped cure cases of prolapsus uteri. These botanicals, along with life-root, black cohosh, fenugreek seed, and that 18 percent alcohol went into Lydia's Compound. And onto the label went claims for relieving the entire gamut of women's peculiar physiological ailments.

Among those seeking to make money from offering customers self-help, temptations arise. Lydia and her sons were not immune. They had worked desperately hard to acquaint women with their product by distributing pamphlets, first in Lynn, then in other New England towns. The first sales significant enough to inscribe in a ledger were made in April 1875, so this self-help symposium celebrates an anniversary. Soon

Daniel Pinkham journeyed to introduce the Vegetable Compound to New York City. He wrote home to brother Will: "I think there is one thing we are missing it on; and that is, not having something on the pamphlets in regard to Kidney Complaints as about half of the people out here are either troubled with Kidney complaints or else think they are. I think you better put something about Kidney complaints of both sexes in very conspicuous type on the first page. . . ."[13]

And so the Pinkham pamphlets began to promote the Compound for kidney complaints of both sexes and for ailments of men's generative organs as well. It was the appeal to women, however, that made the Compound profitable and famous, Lydia's benign face becoming no doubt the best-known feminine visage in America. Since the cut of the trademark was the only illustration of a female that many village newspapers possessed, Lydia now and then appeared as Queen Victoria.[14] The two women had been born in the same year. Indeed, a female pill which competed with the Vegetable Compound was named for Victoria's physician—a brazen act of robbery by a male American nostrum-maker, who further falsely asserted on the pill's wrapper, "Patronized by the Queen."[15]

Daniel Pinkham's attempt to open up a male market is nonetheless instructive. The maker of bottled self-help seldom strays from a prime goal, whatever his other purposes may be: to maximize sales. He has constantly done as Daniel did, observed what potential customers are suffering from in order to frame claims for what his patent medicine can do. The mercenary motive, of course, must never show. Instead, promoters presented themselves as the people's friend, the good samaritan, the ministering angel. But the basic drive for profit was always there. This still holds true in a proprietary medicine climate vastly different from that of a century ago.

In *American Self-Dosage Medicines,* I sought to focus on "the emergence from quackery of American proprietary medicines and their ascent under pressure to successive levels of greater respectability. . . ."[16] While outright quackery has not been subdued, laws regulating drugs and advertising, and developments in science and in the ethical standards of business behavior, have created the modern proprietary industry. Massive in size, it is distinctly restricted in therapeutic scope, its wares confined to treating the symptoms of minor self-limiting ailments and conditions. Yet the time-honored imperative for selling self-help still reigns, to maximize sales. A new confrontation between the proprietary industry and regulatory agencies is now in progress. Central issues relate to the effectiveness of ingredients and the legitimacy of promotional claims. Do modern proprietaries consist of an ounce of physiological efficacy and a pound of placebo? If their claims are not so outrageous as in the nineteenth century, do the explicit and especially the implied promises in their advertising still exceed warrant?

"Just watch television for one evening and judge for yourself," a pharmacist wrote not long ago. "See how many of life's problems are caused by commonly known diseases like 'the blahs,' or see how 'a little blue pill' can save your marriage, or witness how aspirin suddenly has become a sleeping potion, or be amazed at the myriad of psychological and sociological problems that are allegedly the result of 'irregularity.'"[17]

Certainly some current efforts to maximize markets will not survive the Food and Drug Administration's present comprehensive review of over-the-counter drugs and the Federal Trade Commission's efforts to tighten advertising standards.

Another disturbing question has recently been raised—and hotly debated—respecting proprietaries. Has the enormous and unrelenting pressure of their promotion helped persuade the younger generation that drug-taking is a legitimate way of confronting troublesome problems? "Let no one delude himself into thinking," a professor of public health testified before a Senate subcommittee, "there is no nexus between excessive self-medication and use of illegal drugs. Good epidemiologic studies show that parents who use inordinate amounts of medicaments breed children who have a far greater likelihood of using illicit drugs."[18]

From what has been said so far about the sellers of patent medicines, a glimpse of the buyers already has been provided. If they do not keep self-medication diaries, they reveal themselves in other ways. Studying the advertising of successful nostrums affords clues to the motivations of those purchasing patent medicines. Private papers also offer hints. In scanning recently the accumulated papers of a farm family from rural Georgia, I found the collection filled with direct mail nostrum advertising, saved as carefully as letters from cousins in Arkansas. A student of mine has apprised me that a Georgia bishop communicated with the makers of patent medicines he took.[19] Lydia Pinkham was not unique in receiving a vast flood of incoming mail, asking advice and volunteering testimony. Other proprietors also answered their mail, prescribing their remedies over slogans like Lydia's "Yours for Health." Most promoters were less honorable than she with respect to confidentiality, bundling up letters in huge batches, organized by symptom categories, and selling or renting them to other proprietors.[20]

The Pinkham sense of restraint passed on to Lydia's heirs. At some time before the transfer by the family of the company records to the Schlesinger Library of Radcliffe College, the thousands of candid letters written in by inquiring women were removed from the collection.[21] Thus no male eye shall ever see them. One may note a pang of regret that female researchers may not study this rich, lost source of insight into the minds and bodies of women at the end of the nineteenth and beginning of the twentieth century.

What emerges from all these sources, of course, is that life is tough, fraught with tensions and disappointments, with boredom and worries, with minor ailments and major diseases, both of which acquire emotional overlays, while emotional concerns alone can produce distinct physiological symptoms.[22]

Self-help, of course, has a high enough percentage of success to build confidence in the means employed. If the ailment be minor and emotional, the mere act of doing something—anything—may bring relief. Even in more serious conditions, a significant placebo effect comes into play. Almost anything new that is tried helps most arthritic sufferers for a time. If the ailment be minor and self-limited and of short duration, nature achieves the cure for which a nostrum gets the credit. Modern authorities recognize that a large measure of the consumer satisfaction derived from using present-day proprietaries derives from the placebo effect.[23] Even in the gravest diseases, like cancer, some dying patients swear by quacks, parroting the charlatan's assertion that the treatment had done much good and would have cured if begun soon enough.

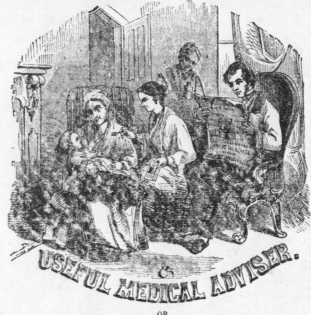

THE

ANNUAL FAMILY

RECEIPT BOOK

& USEFUL MEDICAL ADVISER.

OR

EVERY BODY'S BOOK,

Containing something for Everyone.

NEW-YORK :
A. L. SCOVILL & COMPANY,
GOTHIC HALL, No. 316 BROADWAY.

1854.

Dr. A. Rogers' pamphlet
containing ads and testimonials for his patent medicines.

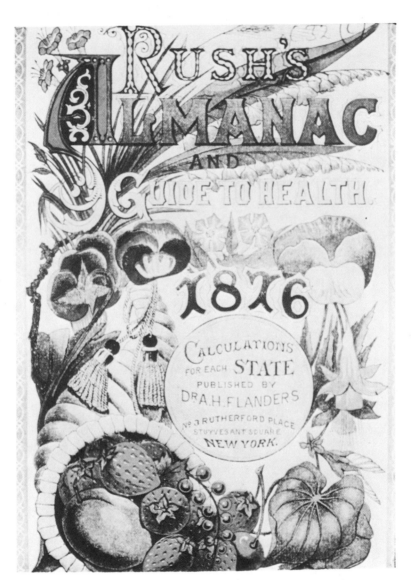

Popular health guide.

In the old days, many patent medicines contained much opium, truly deadening pain. Alcoholic nostrums—some as high as 80 proof—relaxed many users—some with strong temperance convictions—and temporarily gave a more cheerful prospect to gloomy circumstances. From the first, orthodox medical opinion acknowledged the effect of the 18 percent alcohol in Lydia E. Pinkham's Vegetable Compound upon a woman's mood, while not sharing Lydia's confidence in the therapeutic action of her botanicals.[24] Her proclaimed interest in the suffering of women, the promises in her advertising, the cheerful tone of her letters, no doubt her very femaleness, also helped those who dosed themselves with her proprietary. Sales held up even after the pressure of food and drug laws forced a steady retreat from the initial bold and explicit claims upon the label to such simple but subtle recommendations of the Compound "as a vegetable tonic in conditions for which this preparation is adapted."[25]

Many nostrums have recruited legions of faithful users when the ingredients could have had no helpful physiological effects at all. Ardent testimonials, and even testimony in court, supported a diabetes "cure" consisting of the abandonment of insulin in favor of saltpeter dissolved in vinegar. Such praise came from victims whose new mode of treatment already was moving them swiftly toward their graves.[26] Even in the most disastrous circumstances, self-help manages to get a good name.

Americans have been especially impatient about illness. They have wanted something done—and soon—and have been prone to take things into their own hands, *not* consulting physicians, *before* consulting physicians, *while* consulting physicians. This was true in Lydia Pinkham's day, and the attitude continues. A recent behavioral survey, financed by seven federal agencies, spoke of this widespread American trait as "rampant empiricism."[27] Basing decisions on no coherent body of health knowledge, millions of Americans think "anything is worth a try." If orthodox medicine opposes, that does not matter much. Forty-two percent of American adults, the survey revealed, would not be persuaded by almost unanimous expert opinion that a purported "cancer cure" held out false hope. One out of every fifty adults does something virtually every day, acting alone and without a physicians's advice, to move his bowels. One out of eight asserted that he or she would self-medicate, without seeing a doctor, for more than two weeks while treating such symptoms as sore throat, cough, upset stomach, and insomnia.

Three out of four Americans cherish the magical belief that, no matter how sufficient their diets, taking extra vitamins automatically provides more energy and pep. From the ranks of this large segment of the population, stirred by promoters of the more extravagant dietary supplements and operators of health food stores, came a barrage of mail descending upon the last session of the Congress—a barrage said to have been of greater intensity than that provoked by Watergate—in support of a bill that would have gutted the Food and Drug Administration's controls over special dietary wares.[28] The bill swept through the Senate by a ratio of eight to one but remained bottled up in conference committee at the end of the session. The Senate bill, as the Food and Drug Commissioner saw it, was "a charlatan's dream."[29] Senate and House champions of this crusade have collaborated on and introduced into the current Congress another bill, milder in its terms but still affording borderline promoters of dietary wares plenty of elbow room.[30] The FDA, of course, has not been seeking to prevent self-help by resort to vitamins and other special dietary products, but has striven to have them meet rational standards and bear informative labeling.

During the course of history, patent medicines have provided a little help to some of their users by easing minor symptoms of self-limiting ailments, by furnishing a sense of relief through the sheer act of doing something, by encouraging mood. There has been a darker side: the creation of narcotic addicts and alcoholics, the conversion of remediable into incurable ailments because of delay at the futile way-station of self-help. Self-help may not even be a proper term to apply to self-dosage with proprietary medicines. The self has hardly been a free and independent agent under the tremendous, clever pressure of advertising, the main unvarying goal of which has been rather the self-help of the advertiser than the self-help of the suffering citizen belabored to believe that whatever his trouble—from the consumption of yore to the "blahs" of recent date—some commercial pill or potion can produce a cure.

112

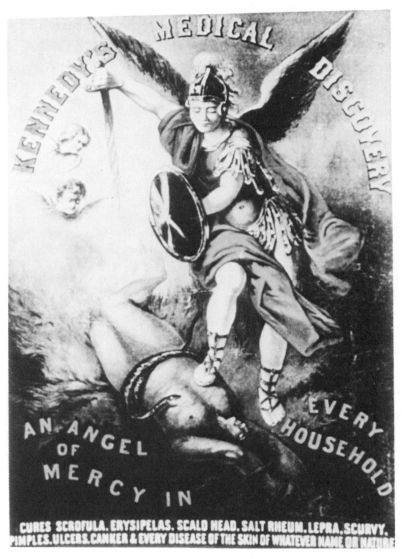

Advertisement for a cure-all household remedy.

"Advertisers and flourishers know perfectly well," wrote an editorialist back in 1871, "that even the gravest and most cautious are to a certain extent touched by their appeals, and that even in the act of denunciation, the most careful often find themselves seduced."[31]

References

[1] Oliver Wendell Holmes, *Medical Essays, 1842–1882* (Boston: Houghton Mifflin Co., 1892), p. 186.

[2] For an example, see Robert B. Shaw, *History of the Comstock Patent Medicine Business and Dr. Morse's Indian Root Pills,* Smithsonian Studies in History and Technology, No. 22 (Washington: Smithsonian Institution Press, 1972).

[3] Grete de Francesco, *The Power of the Charlatan* (New Haven: Yale University Press, 1939), pp. 27–28.

[4] Cited in E.S. Turner, *The Shocking History of Advertising!* (New York: Dutton, 1953), p. 25.

[5] George B. Griffenhagen and James Harvey Young, *Old English Patent Medicines in America,* Contributions from the Museum of History and Technology, paper 10. U.S. National Museum Bulletin 218 (Washington: Smithsonian Institution, 1959), pp. 155–183.

[6] An example is the ointment for the itch advertised in the *Pennsylvania Gazette,* Aug. 19, 1731, by Sarah Read, publisher Benjamin Franklin's mother-in-law.

[7] See Ronald L. Numbers, "Do-It-Yourself the Sectarian Way," in this volume.

[8] The discussion of American patent medicines during their formative period is based on my *The Toadstool Millionaires* (Princeton, N.J.: Princeton University Press, 1961).

[9] Neil Harris, *Humbug, The Art of P.T. Barnum* (Boston: Little, Brown, 1973). Harris does not explicitly point his more general analysis toward patent medicine promotion, as I have done here.

[10] The discussion of Lydia E. Pinkham is based mainly on Robert Collyer Washburn, *The Life and Times of Lydia E. Pinkham* (New York: G.P. Putnam's Sons, 1931); Jean Burton, *Lydia Pinkham Is Her Name* (New York: Farrar, Straus, 1949); and J.H. Young, "Lydia Estes Pinkham," in Edward T. James, ed., *Notable American Women 1607–1950* (Cambridge, Mass.: Belknap Press of Harvard University Press, 1971), III, pp. 71–72. Martha Verbrugge of Cambridge presented a paper on Lydia Pinkham at the 1975 convention of the American Association for the History of Medicine, and Sarah Stage of Williams College is completing a dissertation at Yale University on Mrs. Pinkham.

[11] A retrospective look at this theme may be found in John S. and Robin M. Haller, *The Physician and Sexuality in Victorian America* (Urbana: University of Illinois Press, 1974).

[12] John King, *The American Dispensatory* 8th ed. (Cincinnati: Wilstach, Baldwin & Co., 1870), pp. 78–79, 142–144.

[13] Burton, *Lydia Pinkham Is Her Name*, p. 89.

[14] *Printer's Ink* CXXI (Oct. 5, 1922): 44.

[15] Richard F. Riley, "Caveat Emptor—19th Century American Style," *American Philatelist* LXXXIX (Jan. 1975): 31–34.

[16] James Harvey Young, *American Self-Dosage Medicines, An Historical Perspective* (Lawrence, Kansas: Coronado Press, 1974). The quotation appears on p. xiii.

[17] W. James Bicket, "Autotherapy—'The Future Is Now,'" *Journal of the American Pharmaceutical Association* ns XII (1972): 562.

[18] Testimony of Donald B. Louria, Department of Public Health and Preventive Medicine, New Jersey College of Medicine, July 22, 1971, *Advertising of Proprietary Medicines,* Hearings before the Subcommittee on Monopoly of the Select Committee on Small Business, U.S. Senate, 92nd Congress, 1st session (Washington: U.S. Govt. Printing Ofc., 1971), p. 509.

[19] Hunnicutt Family Papers and Warren A. Candler Papers, Special Collections Department, Robert A. Woodruff Library for Advanced Studies, Emory University, Atlanta, Ga. Mark Bauman called my attention to the letters in Bishop Candler's Papers.

[20] "Strictly Confidential," in Samuel Hopkins Adams, *The Great American Fraud* (Chicago: P.F. Collier, 1906), pp. 142-146.

[21] Conversation with Diane M. Dorsey, Archivist, The Arthur and Elizabeth Schlesinger Library on the History of Women in America, Radcliffe College, Cambridge, Mass. Oct. 8, 1971; Eva Moseley, Curator of Manuscripts, Schlesinger Library, to author, Feb. 18, 1975.

[22] James Harvey Young, "The Persistence of Medical Quackery in America," *American Scientist* LX (1972): 318-326.

[23] Joseph D. Cooper, ed., *The Efficacy of Self-Medication,* Vol. 4, Philosophy and Technology of Drug Assessment, (Washington: Smithsonian Institution, 1973).

[24] *Journal of the American Medical Association* CXII (1939): 2082-2083; E. Lee Strohl, "Ladies of Lynn—Emphasis on One," *Surgery, Gynecology & Obstetrics* CV (1957): 769-775; Oliver Field, Department of Investigation, American Medical Association, to author, July 5, 1960.

[25] From label as of 1933.

[26] James Harvey Young, *The Medical Messiahs* (Princeton, N.J.: Princeton University Press, 1967), pp. 217-238.

[27] *A Study of Health Practices and Opinions* was conducted by National Analysts, Inc., under contract and was published in 1972 by the National Technical Information Service of Springfield, Va.

[28] J.H. Young, "A Threat to Self-Dosing Consumers," *Atlanta Medicine* XLVIII (Dec. 1974): 19, 30; *Atlanta Constitution,* June 25, 1973; *FDC Reports* XXXV (Aug. 6, 1973): 12; (Aug. 13, 1973): T&G 9; XXXVI (Sept. 30, 1974): T&G 9.

[29] Statement by Alexander M. Schmidt, M.D., Commissioner, Food and Drug Administration, before the Subcommittee on Health, Committee on Labor and Public Welfare, U.S. Senate, Aug. 14, 1974.

[30] S. 1692 and H.R. 6807, *Congressional Record,* 94th Congress, 1st session, May 7, 1975, pp. H3818—H3820; May 8, 1975, pp. S7668—S7670. In April 1976 this vitamin bill became law (Public Law 94-278).

[31] "Thoughts on Puffing," *All the Year Round* XXV (1871): 330.

The Contributors

John B. Blake, PH.D. is Chief, History of Medicine Division, National Library of Medicine, Bethesda, Maryland.

James H. Cassedy, PH.D. is a Historian at the National Library of Medicine, Bethesda, Maryland.

Judith Walzer Leavitt, PH.D. is Assistant Professor of the History of Medicine, University of Wisconsin-Madison.

Regina Markell Morantz, PH.D. is Assistant Professor of History, University of Kansas, Lawrence.

Ronald L. Numbers, PH.D. is Associate Professor of the History of Medicine, University of Wisconsin-Madison.

Guenter B. Risse, M.D., PH.D. is Professor and Chairman, Department of the History of Medicine, University of Wisconsin-Madison.

James Harvey Young, PH.D. is Professor of History, Emory University, Atlanta, Georgia.

Index*

*prepared by Lawrence D. Lynch